This report contains the collective views of an international group of experts and does not necessarily represent the decisions or the stated policy of the United Nations Environment Programme, the International Labour Organisation, or the World Health Organization.

Environmental Health Criteria 129

ISOBENZAN

First draft prepared by Dr E.A.H. van Heemstra-Lequin and Dr G.J. van Esch, Netherlands

Published under the joint sponsorship of the United Nations Environment Programme, the International Labour Organisation, and the World Health Organization

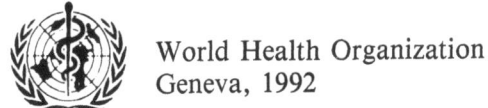

World Health Organization
Geneva, 1992

The **International Programme on Chemical Safety** (IPCS) is a joint venture of the United Nations Environment Programme, the International Labour Organisation, and the World Health Organization. The main objective of the IPCS is to carry out and disseminate evaluations of the effects of chemicals on human health and the quality of the environment. Supporting activities include the development of epidemiological, experimental laboratory, and risk-assessment methods that could produce internationally comparable results, and the development of manpower in the field of toxicology. Other activities carried out by the IPCS include the development of know-how for coping with chemical accidents, coordination of laboratory testing and epidemiological studies, and promotion of research on the mechanisms of the biological action of chemicals.

WHO Library Cataloguing in Publication Data

Isobenzan.

(Environmental health criteria ; 129)

1.Insecticides, Organochlorine - toxicity   2.Environmental exposure
I.Series

ISBN 92 4 157129 2   (NLM Classification: WA 240)
ISSN 0250-863X

©World Health Organization 1991

Publications of the World Health Organization enjoy copyright protection in accordance with the provisions of Protocol 2 of the Universal Copyright Convention. For rights of reproduction or translation of WHO publications, in part or *in toto*, application should be made to the Office of Publications, World Health Organization, Geneva, Switzerland. The World Health Organization welcomes such applications.

The designations employed and the presentation of the material in this publication do not imply the expression of any opinion whatsoever on the part of the Secretariat of the World Health Organization concerning the legal status of any country, territory, city, or area or of its authorities, or concerning the delimitation of its frontiers or boundaries.

The mention of specific companies or of certain manufacturers' products does not imply that they are endorsed or recommended by the World Health Organization in preference to others of a similar nature that are not mentioned. Errors and omissions excepted, the names of proprietary products are distinguished by initial capital letters.

PRINTED IN FINLAND
Vammalan Kirjapaino Oy
92/9012 — VAMMALA — 5500

CONTENTS

ENVIRONMENTAL HEALTH CRITERIA FOR ISOBENZAN

1. SUMMARY AND EVALUATION; CONCLUSIONS AND RECOMMENDATIONS   9

    1.1 Summary and evaluation   9
    1.2 Conclusions and recommendations   11

2. IDENTITY, PHYSICAL AND CHEMICAL PROPERTIES, ANALYTICAL METHODS   12

    2.1 Identity   12
    2.2 Physical and chemical properties   12
    2.3 Conversion factors   13
    2.4 Analytical methods   13

3. SOURCES OF HUMAN AND ENVIRONMENTAL EXPOSURE   15

4. ENVIRONMENTAL TRANSPORT, DISTRIBUTION, AND TRANSFORMATION   16

    4.1 Transport and distribution between media   16
    4.2 Biotransformation   16
        4.2.1 Soil   16
        4.2.2 Water   16

5. ENVIRONMENTAL LEVELS AND HUMAN EXPOSURE   18

    5.1 Environmental levels   18
        5.1.1 Water   18
        5.1.2 Soil   18
        5.1.3 Food   19
            5.1.3.1 Plant products   19
            5.1.3.2 Products of domestic animals   21
            5.1.3.3 Market surveys   22
        5.1.4 Terrestrial and aquatic organisms   22
    5.2 General population exposure   23
    5.3 Occupational exposure   23

6.	KINETICS AND METABOLISM		25
	6.1 Absorption		25
	6.2 Distribution		25
		6.2.1 Rat	25
		6.2.2 Dog	26
		6.2.3 Domestic fowl	27
		6.2.4 Cow	27
	6.3 Metabolic transformation		28
		6.3.1 Vertebrates	28
		6.3.2 Invertebrates	28
		6.3.3 Microorganisms	29
	6.4 Elimination and excretion in expired air, faeces, and urine		29
		6.4.1 Oral administration	29
		6.4.2 Parenteral administration	29
	6.5 Retention and turnover		30
7.	EFFECTS ON LABORATORY MAMMALS AND *IN VITRO* TEST SYSTEMS		31
	7.1 Single exposure		31
		7.1.1 Oral administration	31
		7.1.2 Dermal administration	32
		7.1.3 Parenteral administration	32
		7.1.4 Formulated material	33
		7.1.5 Metabolites	33
	7.2 Short-term exposure		33
		7.2.1 Oral administration	33
		7.2.1.1 Mouse	33
		7.2.1.2 Rat	35
		7.2.1.3 Dog	36
		7.2.2 Dermal administration	37
		7.2.3 Intraperitoneal administration	37
	7.3 Long-term exposure		37
		7.3.1 Rat	37
	7.4 Skin irritation		38
	7.5 Reproductive toxicity, embryotoxicity, and teratogenicity		38
		7.5.1 Mouse	39
		7.5.2 Rat	39
		7.5.3 Dog	39
	7.6 Mutagenicity and related end-points		40
	7.7 Carcinogenicity		40
		7.7.1 Mouse	40

	7.7.2	Rat	40
7.8	Special studies		40
	7.8.1	Biochemical studies	40
	7.8.2	Neurotoxicity	41
	7.8.3	Pharmacological studies	42

8. EFFECTS ON HUMANS ... 43

   8.1 General population exposure ... 43
   8.2 Occupational exposure ... 43

9. EFFECTS ON OTHER ORGANISMS IN THE LABORATORY AND FIELD ... 45

   9.1 Microorganisms ... 45
   9.2 Aquatic organisms ... 45
   9.3 Terrestrial organisms ... 46
      9.3.1 Soil invertebrates ... 46
      9.3.2 Birds ... 46
         9.3.2.1 Acute toxicity ... 46
         9.3.2.2 Short-term toxicity ... 46
   9.4 Population and ecosystem effects ... 47
      9.4.1 Soil microorganisms ... 47
      9.4.2 Soil invertebrates ... 48

REFERENCES ... 49

RESUME ET EVALUATION; CONCLUSIONS ET RECOMMANDATIONS ... 55

RESUMEN Y EVALUACION; CONCLUSIONES Y RECOMENDACIONES ... 59

WHO TASK GROUP ON ENVIRONMENTAL HEALTH CRITERIA FOR ISOBENZAN

Members

Dr L.A. Albert, Xalapa, Veracruz, Mexico

Dr V. Benes, Department of Toxicology and Reference Laboratory, Institute of Hygiene and Epidemiology, Prague, Czechoslovakia

Dr S. Dobson, Institute of Terrestrial Ecology, Monks Wood Experimental Station, Huntingdon, United Kingdom

Dr S.K. Kashyap, National Institute of Occupational Health, Ahmedabad, India

Dr Y.I. Kundiev, Research Institute of Labour Hygiene and Occupational Diseases, Kiev, USSR *(Vice-Chairman)*

Dr Y. Osman, Ministry of Health, Riyadh, Saudi Arabia

Dr H. Spencer, Office of Pesticides Programs, US Environmental Protection Agency, Washington, D.C., USA *(Chairman)*

Dr G.J. van Esch, Bilthoven, Netherlands *(Joint Rapporteur)*

Dr E.A.H. van Heemstra-Lequin, Laren, Netherlands *(Joint Rapporteur)*

Dr C. Winder, National Institute of Occupational Health and Safety, Forest Lodge, New South Wales, Australia

Secretariat

Dr K.W. Jager, International Programme on Chemical Safety, World Health Organization, Geneva, Switzerland *(Secretary)*

Ms B. Labarthe, International Register of Potentially Toxic Chemicals, United Nations Environment Programme, Geneva, Switzerland

Dr T.K. Ng, Office of Occupational Health, World Health Organization, Geneva, Switzerland

NOTE TO READERS OF THE CRITERIA DOCUMENTS

Every effort has been made to present information in the criteria documents as accurately as possible without unduly delaying their publication. In the interest of all users of the environmental health criteria documents, readers are kindly requested to communicate any errors that may have occurred to the Manager of the International Programme on Chemical Safety, World Health Organization, Geneva, Switzerland, in order that they may be included in corrigenda.

* * *

A detailed data profile and a legal file can be obtained from the International Register of Potentially Toxic Chemicals, Palais des Nations, 1211 Geneva 10, Switzerland (Telephone No. 7988400 or 7985850).

ENVIRONMENTAL HEALTH CRITERIA FOR ISOBENZAN

A WHO Task Group on Environmental Health Criteria for Isobenzan met at the World Health Organization, Geneva, from 23 to 27 July 1990. Dr K.W. Jager welcomed the participants on behalf of Dr M. Mercier, Manager of the IPCS, and the three IPCS cooperating organizations (UNEP/ILO/WHO). The Task Group reviewed and revised the draft document and made an evaluation of the risks for human health and the environment from exposure to isobenzan.

The first draft of this document was prepared in cooperation between Dr E.A.H. van Heemstra-Lequin and Dr G.J. van Esch of the Netherlands. Dr van Esch prepared the second draft, incorporating the comments received following circulation of the first draft to the IPCS contact points for Environmental Health Criteria documents. Dr K.W. Jager and Dr P.G. Jenkins, both members of the IPCS Central Unit, were responsible for the scientific content and technical editing, respectively.

The assistance of Shell in making available to the IPCS and the Task Group its proprietary toxicological information on its products is gratefully acknowledge. This allowed the Task Group to make their evaluation on the basis of more complete data.

The efforts of all who helped in the preparation and finalization of the document are gratefully acknowledged.

1. SUMMARY AND EVALUATION; CONCLUSIONS AND RECOMMENDATIONS

1.1 Summary and evaluation

As far as is known, isobenzan, an organochlorine insecticide, was only manufactured during the period 1958-1965. It was used from existing stocks for several years thereafter. At present, the only major sources of exposure are believed to be the original waste-disposal sites of industrial wastes or dredgings from contaminated sediments.

After isobenzan is applied to soil, a rapid initial loss occurs, after which the remaining compound decays at a much slower rate. It persists in soil from 2 to 7 years depending on the type of soil. Under laboratory conditions isobenzan decomposes in surface water within a few weeks when exposed to natural or artificial light.

Soil, ground water, and surface water from polders built up using sediment contaminated with organochlorines, including chlorinated cyclodiene compounds, still contained minor residues of isobenzan some years later. In 1979-1980, no isobenzan was detected (detection limit: 0.01 mg/kg dry weight) in the sediment of rivers in the Netherlands. Following soil treatment, residues in crops are usually low (below 0.05 mg/kg crop), but higher levels may be found in some root crops (up to 0.2 mg/kg in carrots). In market surveys conducted during the time of the agricultural use of isobenzan, no residues were detected in the food items analysed (less than 0.01 mg/kg).

After cattle were allowed to graze pastures treated with isobenzan, the resultant daily products contained residues of the insecticide. Two samples of butter contained 0.07 and 0.15 mg isobenzan/kg product, while the levels in whole milk were 0.005 to 0.07 mg/kg. Dried milk, however, contained only 0.005 mg/kg. During the processing of dairy products, up to 50% of the residue was lost, depending on the type of treatment.

No data are available on the levels of isobenzan in the blood or adipose tissue of the general population. Operators exposed to isobenzan in manufacturing and formulation plants had mean whole blood levels of up to 0.041 mg/litre. In whole blood samples of people living in the neighbourhood of one plant, the concentration of isobenzan was below the limit of detection (0.001 mg/litre).

Summary and Evaluation; Conclusions and Recommendations

Isobenzan is readily absorbed through the gastrointestinal wall and is transported in the blood as the unchanged compound. Hydrophilic metabolites are formed, one of which has been identified as isobenzan lactone. Isobenzan accumulates in the tissues and organs of rats and dogs in the following order: fat > liver = muscle > brain > blood. The tissue concentrations of female rats are generally higher than those of males, especially in body fat. The biological half-life in body fat was found to be 10.9 days in male rats and 16.6 days in female rats. A female canine pup, whose blood contained 0.09 mg isobenzan/litre, showed convulsions 15 days after birth. The pup had only fed on the milk of its mother, a Beagle hound that had been dosed with isobenzan and whose milk contained 0.7 mg/litre. Similar effects on pups were seen in a rat reproduction study. Isobenzan is excreted via the milk of cows.

Mosquito larvae and soil fungi metabolize isobenzan in the same way as vertebrates, yielding isobenzan lactone as a metabolite.

Isobenzan is very persistent in the environment and bioaccumulates. It is highly toxic to fish, shrimps, and birds. In the Netherlands, the country where isobenzan was manufactured, residues in the eggs of terns living along the Dutch coast ranged up to 0.45 mg/kg (mean, 0.09 mg/kg), while mean residues in mussels and fish were 0.05 mg/kg in 1965. Earthworm numbers were found to be reduced in field plots treated with isobenzan at 2 kg/ha. Nitrification was reduced, with a consequent increase in inorganic nitrogen, in soils treated with isobenzan in the field at 1 kg/ha, although laboratory studies showed no effect on nitrification at doses equivalent to 250 g/ha.

The acute toxicity of isobenzan to mammals is high, both by the oral and percutaneous routes. The mode of action of its toxicity is an overstimulation of the central nervous system, resulting in convulsions. The acute toxicity of formulations of isobenzan reflects the percentage of active ingredient present.

Isobenzan is not a skin irritant, but some formulated products may cause irritation.

Limited short- and long-term oral studies in mice, rats, and dogs have shown that isobenzan may cause histological changes of the classical type of organochlorine intoxication in the liver. In a long-term rat study, a no-observed-effect level of 5 mg/kg diet (approximately 0.25 mg/kg body weight) was determined, and in a 2-year dog study the no-observed-adverse-effect level (NOAEL) was 0.025 mg/kg body weight.

A one-generation reproduction study in rats indicated a NOAEL of 0.1 mg/kg diet (approximately 0.005 mg/kg body weight). At a level of 1 mg/kg diet (approximately 0.05 mg/kg body weight) the survival of pups decreased.

No teratogenicity or mutagenicity studies have been reported.

No carcinogenic potential was demonstrated in a 2-year oral study on rats and in an oral study on mice, but these studies were inadequate to evaluate carcinogenicity.

The toxicological data base for isobenzan is incomplete. In general, the quality of the data is considered to be poor by today's standards and inadequate for an evaluation of the hazards to human health or the environment.

Data on exposed humans are limited to studies on workers in a factory in the Netherlands during the manufacture and formulation of isobenzan and related "chlorinated cyclodiene insecticides". No cases of skin irritation were reported. In several cases of intoxication, convulsions occurred but the changes in the EEG pattern were reversible. The intoxication threshold level (for convulsions) was estimated to be 0.015 mg isobenzan/litre blood, and the biological half-life of isobenzan in human blood was estimated to be of the order of 2.8 years.

1.2 Conclusions and recommendations

Isobenzan is highly toxic and very persistent. The available information on the hazards of isobenzan is incomplete, but is, nevertheless, sufficient to indicate that the hazard it poses to those who handling it and to the environment is such that no human or environmental exposure to this substance, used either as an insecticide or for any other purpose, should be allowed.

2. IDENTITY, PHYSICAL AND CHEMICAL PROPERTIES, ANALYTICAL METHODS

2.1 Identity

Chemical formula $C_9H_4OCl_8$

Chemical structure
and spatial
configuration

Chemical names 1,3,4,5,6,7,8,8-octachloro-4,7-methylene-3a,4,7,7a-tetrahydro-isobenzofuran

Common synonyms BAS-4402; CP 14957; ENT-25 545; OMS-206; OMS-618; SD-4402; WL 1650; preparation 948

Common trade name Telodrin (technical product), Omtan

Purity (technical) not less than 95% (w/w)

RTECS registry
number PC1225000

CAS registry number 297-78-9

2.2 Physical and chemical properties

Some physical and chemical properties of isobenzan are given in Table 1.

Table 1. Some physical and chemical properties of isobenzan

Physical state	crystalline powder
Colour	whitish to light brown
Odour	mild "chemical" odour
Relative molecular mass	411.73
Melting point (°C)	120-122
Flash point	non-flammable
Explosion limits	non-explosive
Relative density	1.87
Vapour pressure (20 °C)	6.7×10^{-4} Pa (5×10^{-6} mmHg)
Solubility in water	practically insoluble
Solubility in organic solvents	slightly soluble in kerosene and ethanol; soluble in acetone, benzene, toluene, xylene, heavy aromatic naphtha, and ethyl ether
Stability	relatively stable to acids; dehydrochlorination may occur under strong alkaline conditions

2.3 Conversion factors

1 ppm = 17 mg/m³ at 20 °C
1 mg/m³ = 0.06 ppm at 20 °C

2.4 Analytical methods

Analytical methods for the extraction, preparation, and determination of residues of isobenzan in crops, animal products, and soil using gas-liquid chromatography with electron-capture detection have been described in detail by Elgar (1966) and Anon (1974). The limit of determination is 0.01 mg/kg.

Kadoum (1968) described a rapid micromethod of sample clean-up for gas-chromatographic analysis of isobenzan in ground water, soil, and plant and animal extracts, using activated silica gel of high purity. The percentage recovery was from 90% to 99% depending on the quantity of eluate (305 v/v benzene in hexane) used. The limit of determination in soil and plant or animal tissue was 0.01 mg/kg and in water was 0.01 µg/litre.

Suzuki et al. (1974) analysed different types of pesticides in extracts from crops or soil and separated them into a number of groups by column chromatography (prior to thin-layer chromatography) to obtain a systematic identification and determination of these compounds. Silica gel was used for column chromatography and thin-layer plates. For gas chromatographic separation, glass columns packed with different absorbents were used. Electron capture detection and a ^{63}Ni source were used for the determination.

An advanced residue method, i.e. automated glass capillary gas chromatography with electron-capture detection, was described by Tuinstra & Traag (1979) for use with soil, vegetable material, milk fat, and feed stuffs.

Wegman & Hofstee (1982) used capillary gas chromatography with electron-capture determination for soil and river sediment samples.

The analysis of isobenzan in blood can be carried out according to the method of Richardson et al. (1967) using gas-liquid chromatography with electron-capture determination. The method is sufficiently sensitive to detect isobenzan levels of less than 1 µg/litre blood.

Confirmation tests should be carried out using an appropriate method (Anon, 1974).

3. SOURCES OF HUMAN AND ENVIRONMENTAL EXPOSURE

Telodrin was the registered trademark for the chlorinated cyclodiene insecticide isobenzan. Isobenzan was only manufactured by Shell during the period 1958-1965, but it was used for several years thereafter from existing stocks. The major sources of exposure at present appear to be the original waste disposal sites of industrial wastes or dredged muds from contaminated areas.

4. ENVIRONMENTAL TRANSPORT, DISTRIBUTION, AND TRANSFORMATION

4.1 Transport and distribution between media

The environmental transport of isobenzan was investigated in a slow sand filtration system used for the purification of ground water. The first filter consisted of gravel and the second of sand. Isobenzan was applied to the inlet water at a concentration of 1-10 µg/litre for 2 consecutive weeks. Fifty days elapsed after the isobenzan treatment before it was no longer detectable in the outstream (Bauer, 1972).

4.2 Biotransformation

4.2.1 Soil

In a study by Bowman et al. (1965), the behaviour of isobenzan in soil was investigated in laboratory tests. Eight types of soil were used ranging from sand to sandy clay, the percentage of sand varying from 93 to 56% and the percentage of clay from 4 to 35%. Following percolation with hexane, the percentage of isobenzan in the eluate fraction was shown to decrease with increasing content of clay in the soil (starting at about 30% clay). Except in the case of sand with a high organic matter content (6-19%), no isobenzan was recovered from the dry soils after 4-8 days of exposure at 45 °C. When the soils were moistened with water and exposed at 45 °C for 4 days, degradation was markedly diminished, with the exception of the sand with high organic matter.

After isobenzan is applied to soil (chalky loam, sandy loam, and peat), a rapid initial loss occurs, probably due to sublimation. The remaining compound then decays at a much lower rate, probably having been adsorbed onto soil particles (Elgar, 1966).

The persistence of isobenzan in soil (95% disappearance) is 2-7 years (average 4 years) following an average dosage of 0.25-1 kg isobenzan/ha (Edwards, 1965).

4.2.2 Water

When river water (pH 7.3) treated with 10 µg isobenzan/litre was kept at room temperature in closed glass containers and exposed to natural and artificial light, 25% of the isobenzan remained after one week and 10% after 2 weeks. After the fourth week, no isobenzan was detectable (detection limit: 50 ng/litre) (Eichelberger & Lichtenberg, 1971).

5. ENVIRONMENTAL LEVELS AND HUMAN EXPOSURE

5.1 Environmental levels

5.1.1 Water

During the period 1969-1977, 1826 samples of surface water, ground water, and rain water were taken at 99 sampling sites all over the Netherlands, with special emphasis on the Rivers Rhine and Meuse. Isobenzan was not present at measurable concentrations in any of the samples (Wegman & Greve, 1980).

Soil samples were taken in 1977 to depths of 1-7 m from a polder near Rotterdam that had been filled with material dredged from the Rotterdam harbours between 1959 and 1976. In the ground water, released from the samples by pressure, the concentration of isobenzan in samples obtained from depths of 1, 3, and 5 m was less than 0.05 µg/litre. The concentrations in those from depths of 2 and 7 m were 0.21 and 0.07 µg/litre, respectively. The surface water taken from the drainage system of the polder contained 0.03 µg/litre. Most of the isobenzan in the polder was bound to solids, the ratio of bound to dissolved isobenzan being over 11 000 to 1 (Kerdijk, 1981).

When 60 samples of water from 19 rivers and their estuaries collected in Japan in 1974 were analysed for isobenzan, none was detected (detection limit: < 0.1 µg/litre) (Japanese Environmental Agency, 1975).

5.1.2 Soil

In a study by Elgar (1966), chalky loam, sandy loam, and peat were treated with 0.5 kg isobenzan/ha (as emulsifiable concentrate) once in 1961 or by three annual applications in 1961-1963. About 15% of the initial residue remained after one year. More than half this amount was still present 2 years later (Table 2).

In a Dutch monitoring programme, 145 sediment samples were taken by dredge at 36 sampling sites in tributaries of the Rhine River, Western Scheldt, and in some harbour basins of Rotterdam during 1979-1980. None of the samples contained isobenzan (the detection limit was 0.01 mg/kg soil on a dry weight basis) (Wegman & Hofstee, 1982).

Sixty samples of bottom deposit from 19 rivers and their estuaries in Japan collected in 1974 did not contain any isobenzan (detection limit: 0.01 mg/kg) (Japanese Environmental Agency, 1975).

Table 2. Residues of isobenzan in 3 soil types after treatment with 0.5 kg isobenzan/ha

Soil type	Years of treatment	Time of sampling						
		Spring 1961	Autumn 1961	Spring 1962	Autumn 1962	Spring[a] 1963	Autumn 1963	Spring 1964
Chalky loam	1961	1.1	0.6	0.6	0.3	0.2	0.2	0.2
	1961, 1962, 1963			1.4	0.7	0.3/0.9	0.5	0.3
Sandy loam	1961	0.6	0.2	0.1	0.1	0.1	0.1	0.2
	1961, 1962, 1963			0.5	0.3	0.2/0.9	0.4	0.3
Peat soil	1961	4.2	0.3	0.2	0.2	0.3	0.3	0.3
	1961, 1962, 1963			1.2	0.7	0.2/1.6	1.1	0.5

[a] The two values represent residues before and after re-spraying.

5.1.3 Food

5.1.3.1 Plant products

Residue data, resulting from both foliar and soil treatment, for a variety of crops have been reported (Shell, 1964).

a) Residues in crops: Foliar treatment

The magnitude of residues found on foliage or fruit is affected by a number of factors. Crops having a large volume but a small surface area tend to start off with a low concentration of isobenzan. When crops have a rough (peach) or waxy (blackcurrant, cabbage) surface, isobenzan appears to be less readily removed by weathering than it is from smooth-skinned crops like tomatoes.

The rate of growth of the edible part of the crop is a consistently significant factor, as is the application rate and concentration. There is no evidence that isobenzan is translocated or absorbed by plants and the rates of dissipation can be explained by weathering of surface deposits, with some adsorption by cuticular fats retarding this process. The period after the last application required for the residue level to fall to below 0.05 mg/kg product varies from 14 to 65 days, depending on the factors mentioned above.

Once a crop has been harvested, the residues present may be further reduced or eliminated before consumption by various subsequent processes. Washing can remove 60% of isobenzan residues on broccoli. Isobenzan is removed when fruit and vegetables (such as tomatoes) are processed to produce juice. Canning and freezing processes (involving washing or blanching) also reduce residue levels. Peeling of fruits (such as peaches) and discarding outer leaves of vegetables (cabbage and lettuce) reduce the residue levels significantly. In the case of tobacco, substantial quantities of isobenzan are lost during both the curing and smoking. Cottonseed has very low levels of residues (of the order of 0.01 mg/kg product) and the major part is found in the crude oil after processing (Shell, 1964).

In 1964, cotton was treated up to 12 times with Telodrin dust or emulsifiable concentrate at a dose of up to 350 g isobenzan/ha in Guatemala, Mexico, and Nicaragua, and the seeds were harvested 17 days after the last treatment. The cotton seed oil contained isobenzan residues of < 0.05 mg/kg (Elgar, 1965; Hughes, 1965).

Isobenzan residues of less than 0.05-1.5 mg/kg were found in tobacco leaves grown in Australia during the period 1961-1964. Cigarettes contained 0.2-0.3 mg/kg and pipe tobacco 0.06 mg/kg (Buick, 1964).

b) Residues in crops resulting from soil treatment

When potatoes (in India and the United Kingdom) and sweet potatoes (in South Africa) were grown in soil treated before planting in 1964 with Telodrin dust or emulsifiable concentrate at up to 3 kg isobenzan/ha or treated three times with Telodrin emulsifiable concentrate at 200 g isobenzan/ha, the residues were near the limit of detection (0.05 mg/kg crop) (Murphy & Standen, 1964; Buick, 1965; Buick & Cole, 1965).

In the United Kingdom, chalky loam, sandy loam, and peat were treated with diluted 15% Telodrin emulsifiable concentrate at a level of 0.5 kg isobenzan/ha. This was immediately incorporated by harrow and, directly after, the plots were sown with cabbage, carrot, onion, and sugar beet seed. Potatoes and celery were planted at a later date. The plots were treated either in 1961 only or in 1961, 1962, and 1963. Residues were found in crops grown in both loam soils, but not in those grown in peat, and only in root crops (at a maximum of 0.05 mg/kg crop) after treatment in 1961. The residues did not increase markedly with annual retreatment, the maximum concentration found being 0.08 mg/kg in carrots (Elgar, 1966).

c) Residues in crops resulting from contaminated soils

Crops and the soil in which they had been grown were sampled at harvest in 1976 from Dutch polders that had been built up during 1967-1969 with sediments dredged from the River Rhine and from a harbour basin near a pesticide manufacturing plant. No residues of isobenzan were detected in onions, brussel sprouts, or potatoes (detection limit: 0.01 mg/kg), whereas carrots contained residues of up to 0.09 mg/kg. The corresponding soil samples contained isobenzan residues of between 0.01 and 3.5 mg/kg (dry weight basis). The ratio of the concentration in carrots to that in soil, both calculated on a dry weight basis, was 0.26 (Wegman et al., 1981).

5.1.3.2 Products of domestic animals

Pasture in Venezuela was treated with isobenzan at an average dosage rate of 300 g/ha, and cattle were reintroduced 3-6 months later. Analysis of the dairy products showed two samples of butter containing residues of 0.07 and 0.15 mg/kg, respectively. In milk, the residues ranged from 0.005 to 0.07 mg/kg, while dried milk contained negligible residues (0.005 mg/kg) (Standen & Elgar, 1965).

Heat treatment of various dairy products manufactured from milk containing 0.8 mg isobenzan/kg (18 mg/kg on fat basis) was found to cause residue losses. Between 40% and 50% of the residues were destroyed in evaporated milk and 10-20% of the residues during processing of the milk for dry whole milk (Stemp & Liska, 1966).

No residues of isobenzan could be detected in chicken meat after white meat containing 0.2 mg/kg or dark meat containing 0.5 mg/kg had been cooked (McCaskey et al., 1968).

In Victoria, Australia, in 1963, dairy pasture was sprayed with 140 g isobenzan/ha and left for 3 weeks before dairy cattle were reintroduced. Within 2 days, toxic symptoms (circling, rolling of eyes, salivation, convulsions) were observed in dairy cattle that had consumed treated grass. Deaths occurred in cattle and calves and in cats, rabbits, poultry, and dogs. A 10-month old baby, fed on milk from the cows, developed an illness characterized by irritability and persistent crying. Milk from one cow with signs of intoxication had an isobenzan level of 1 mg/litre. Analysis of isobenzan residues in farm milk (representing milk from many cows) ranged up to 5 mg/litre, although most values were in the range of 0.05 to 0.2 mg/litre. Residues of isobenzan were still present in some milk samples 14 months later. Isobenzan was also detected in cow adipose tissue (10 mg/kg), cat liver (4.5 mg/kg), and calf liver (7.5 mg/kg). Isobenzan levels in surface water used by the cattle were very low (0.0002 mg/litre) (Shell, 1963).

5.1.3.3 Market surveys

Food items covering the important constituents of the local diet (e.g., potatoes, rice, wheat, onions, different types of beans, fruit, beef, lamb, milk, cheese, ground-nut products, maize, and sugar cane) were collected in Venezuela (1966), Mexico (1967), Nicaragua (1967), Spain (1967), and India (1968). Residues of isobenzan in these products were below the limit of detection (0.01 mg/kg) (Bull & Marlow, 1967; Bull & Ramsden, 1967; Elgar & Holland, 1967; Marlow et al., 1968; Mathews, 1969).

Isobenzan was not detected in market-basket surveys conducted by the Food and Drug Administration in the USA during the period 1980-1990 (Burse, 1990, personal communication to the IPCS).

Cured tobacco from Costa Rica contained 1.3 mg isobenzan/kg (Mathews & Cole, 1966).

5.1.4 Terrestrial and aquatic organisms

Fish, mussels, and the eggs of various species of tern were collected along the north coast of the Netherlands and analysed for residues of chlorinated hydrocarbon insecticides. The mean isobenzan residues in eggs were 0.09 mg/kg (range, 0.02-0.45 mg/kg) in 1965 and 0.06 mg/kg (range, 0.02-0.12 mg/kg) in 1966. The mean residues in composite samples of fish (sprat, juvenile herring, and sand eel) were 0.05 mg/kg (range, 0.04-0.07 mg/kg) in 1965 and 0.02 mg/kg (range, 0.01-0.05 mg/kg) in 1966. Mussels *(Mytilus edulis)* sampled in 1966 did not contain any residues of isobenzan (detection level: 0.003 mg/kg), but mussels sampled at one particular place in 1965 contained 0.11 mg/kg (Koeman et al., 1967, 1968).

Residues in the livers of sandwich terns found dead in the Dutch Wadden Sea during the summers of 1965 and 1966 amounted to as much as 3.8 mg/kg isobenzan (average, approximately 0.75 mg/kg) (Koeman et al., 1967).

Sixty samples of fish and shellfish collected in 19 rivers and their sea estuaries in Japan in 1974 contained no isobenzan (detection limit: 0.005 mg/kg) (Japanese Environmental Agency, 1975).

5.2 General population exposure

A housing estate of about 800 houses and public buildings was built directly on a 4-m thick layer of harbour sludge in the Netherlands in 1983. The area was raised during the period 1962-1964 by sludge originating from about 20 harbour basins in Rotterdam and the industrial area around the Nieuwe Waterweg. In the sludge, organic solvents, polyaromatic hydrocarbons, heavy metals, and chlorinated cyclodiene insecticides including isobenzan were detected. One-third of the soil samples collected in the gardens (71 locations), 0-40 cm below the surface, contained chlorinated cyclodiene insecticides with a mean concentration of 1.2 mg/kg and a maximum concentration of 19.5 mg/kg dry weight (Van Wijnen & Stijkel, 1988).

From the residue data presented in section 5.1.3, it appears that exposure of the general population via food was very low at the time when isobenzan was used agriculturally. Exposure from environmental sources must also have been minor. For example, the concentration of isobenzan in the blood of 10 people living in the vicinity of an isobenzan formulation plant in Venezuela was below the limit of determination (0.001 mg/litre) (Davies, 1966a,b).

5.3 Occupational exposure

In a study carried out in 1965-1968 at a formulation plant in Venezuela, 229 blood samples were taken from operators formulating isobenzan and related chlorinated hydrocarbon insecticides. The concentrations of isobenzan in blood fluctuated during this period due to variations in the formulations being prepared at the plant. The mean concentrations in whole blood ranged from 0.004 to 0.033 mg/litre, the maximum concentration being 0.045 mg/litre (Davies, 1966a,b; Crabtree, 1968).

Isobenzan levels in the range of < 0.002 to 0.041 mg/litre were found in the blood of operators at a manufacturing and formulation plant in the Netherlands (Jager, 1970).

6. KINETICS AND METABOLISM

6.1 Absorption

In studies using everted sacs of rat ileum, colloidal solutions and dispersions of isobenzan labelled with ^{14}C were absorbed through the intestinal wall. The maximum uptake occurred in the middle segment of the ileum (Hathway, 1965).

Following an oral dose of ^{14}C-isobenzan, only a small proportion (< 10%) of the label was found in the thoracic lymph duct, the remainder being in the hepatic portal blood (Hathway, 1965).

6.2 Distribution

Isobenzan is approximately 4000 times more soluble in rabbit serum than in water, and it has been shown that, during transport in the blood of rats and rabbits, isobenzan is associated with some serum proteins (albumin and α-globulin in the rabbit and albumins in the rat) and with constituents of the red blood cell, mainly haemoglobin. The ratio of the distribution of the insecticide between plasma and cells was shown to be approximately 2:1, this ratio remaining constant at different intervals after administration and at different concentrations. Gas chromatography showed that unchanged isobenzan was transported in the blood (Moss & Hathway, 1964; Hathway, 1965).

6.2.1 Rat

In an extensive study, Carworth Farm rats were fed diets containing isobenzan (96%) (5, 15.9, or 25 mg/kg) for periods of 44 to 224 days followed by a control diet for periods of up to 64 days. Analyses of tissues at several intervals during feeding showed the concentrations of isobenzan to be in the following order: fat > liver = muscle > brain > blood. Concentrations in females were higher than those in the males, especially in the fat. There was a significant correlation between the concentration of isobenzan in blood and in other organs, plausibly attributed to a dynamic equilibrium. The biological half-life in body fat was 10.9 days in male rats and 16.6 days in female rats (Robinson & Richardson, 1963).

When male and female rats were given a single intravenous injection of ^{14}C-isobenzan (15 µg/kg body weight), the radioactivity in the blood of males 48 h later was 0.04% of the applied dose and in females was 0.37%. The radioactivity in the organs and tissues ranged between 0.01 and approximately 1.5% of the applied dose, concentrations being lower in females than in males. In abdominal fat, the concentrations were 19.2% in males and 26.6% in females and, in muscle, 12.3% and 9.3%, respectively. The concentration in subcutaneous fat was about half of that in abdominal fat (Kaul et al., 1970).

Isobenzan rapidly crosses the placental barrier in pregnant rats. Labelled isobenzan was found in fetal blood within 5 min of an intravenous administration into the ear vein of the mother (Hathway, 1965).

Fetuses removed by caesarean section from Carworth Farm rats fed a dietary isobenzan concentration of 5 mg/kg in a reproduction study carried out by Chambers (1962a,b) (section 7.5.2) contained 0.1-0.13 mg isobenzan/kg tissue (Stevenson, 1964).

6.2.2 Dog

In a study by (Worden, 1969), groups of six Scottish terriers (males and females) were given daily isobenzan doses of 0.025 or 0.1 mg/kg body weight by gavage for 2 years (section 7.2.1.3). At the end of the study the distribution of isobenzan in the tissues was examined, and the concentration was highest in body fat and least in blood (Table 3). There was a significant correlation between the concentrations in blood and those in other tissues. The storage ratio (concentration in body fat/concentration in diet) did not show any significant differences between the sexes or between the two dose levels.

Table 3. Mean concentrations (mg/kg) of isobenzan in tissues of dogs dosed orally with isobenzan for 2 years

Dose	Fat	Muscle	Liver	Brain	Blood
0.025 mg/kg body weight	2.9	0.25	1.2	0.2	0.02
0.1 mg/kg body weight	9.5	0.8	4.2	0.4	0.04

The first litter from a female Beagle hound dosed with 0.08 mg isobenzan/kg body weight per day (section 7.5.3) consisted of one male, one female, and one still-born male. The concentrations of isobenzan in the brain, liver, muscle, heart, and kidneys of the still-born pup were below 0.2 mg/kg, with the liver containing the highest level of 0.16 mg/kg. The female pup, which only fed on the mother's milk, showed convulsions 15 days after birth and was killed at 17 days of age. The blood contained 0.09 mg isobenzan per kg and the urine 0.02 mg/kg. The concentrations in organs and tissues were less than 1 mg/kg, the highest levels being in muscle (0.94 mg/kg), liver (0.65 mg/kg), and fat (0.48 mg/kg). The milk from the mother contained 0.7 mg/litre as whole milk and 3.4 mg/kg on a fat basis. The remaining pup showed no ill effects. Four males and two females in further litters also showed no ill effects (Brown & Richardson, 1964).

6.2.3 Domestic fowl

In a study by McCaskey et al. (1968), six Leghorn hens received, in a gelatin capsule on each of 5 days, an amount of isobenzan (94% purity) equivalent to 10-15 mg/kg of the average weight of daily feed consumed. Eggs were collected on days 2-8, and the hens were killed 3 days after the last dose. Residues in tissues and eggs are given in Table 4.

Table 4. Concentrations of residues (mg/kg products) in tissues and eggs of hens dosed orally with isobenzan

Tissue	Residue concentration (mg/kg)
Abdominal fat	10.6
White meat	0.2 (on fat basis: 3.4)
Dark meat	0.5 (on fat basis: 4.3)
Egg yolk	0.1 on day 4; 0.4 on day 5; 0.5 on day 7 0.7 on day 8

6.2.4 Cow

Three Jersey cows were fed for 28 days at concentrations of technical isobenzan of 0, 0.005, or 0.02 mg/kg in their daily ration (average ration, 20 kg per cow). Residues found in the milk of the cow fed 0.005 mg/kg increased from 0.4 µg/litre to 2 µg/litre at the end of the feeding period and decreased rapidly thereafter. Higher residues of up to 7.7 µg/litre were present in the milk from the cow fed 0.02 mg/kg, which decreased to 1.5 µg/litre whole milk 10 weeks after the last day of dosing (Hardee et al., 1964).

Following the consumption of feed contaminated with relatively low concentrations of isobenzan, the concentration in milk rose rapidly within a few hours to days, levelling off at a plateau characteristic for each concentration in the diet. The average milk/diet ratio for isobenzan was 0.4 to 0.5 for feeding levels of 0.005 to 0.02 mg/kg diet (Biehl & Buck, 1987).

In a study by Bishop & Huber (1964), four groups of three lactating Holstein cows were fed 0, 0.02, 0.06, or 0.15 mg isobenzan/kg (corresponding to 0.47, 1.38, or 3.38 mg/cow per day) in their daily ration for 90 days. The concentrations in the milk were directly proportional to the dietary level. Increases in concentration were noted during the entire treatment period for the 0.06- and 0.15-mg/kg feeding levels, reaching 0.033 and 0.071 mg/litre of milk. Trace amounts (up to 0.008 mg/litre) were found in the milk from cows fed 0.02 mg/kg. At the highest dose, residues of 0.016 mg/litre were still present in the milk 60 days after treatment, while in the groups fed 0.06 and 0.02 mg/kg, the residues were then negligible. Residues in fat from biopsies taken 88 days after the treatment finished reflected the exposure levels, being 0.11, 0.26, and 0.53 mg/kg tissue for the three levels.

6.3 Metabolic transformation

6.3.1 Vertebrates

The radioactive residue present in the urine and faeces of rats treated with a single intravenous injection of ^{14}C-isobenzan consisted of a hydrophilic metabolite that, after hydrolysis, gave isobenzan lactone (Kaul et al., 1970).

It is probable that both chlorine atoms on the tetrahydrofuran ring are first replaced by hydroxyl groups. The resulting "acetale", an unstable intermediate, is converted to the gamma-lactone (Korte, 1967) (Fig. 1).

6.3.2 Invertebrates

Mosquito larvae (*Aedes aegypti*) metabolize isobenzan, labelled with ^{14}C in the hexachloropentane ring or at the 1,3 position, to

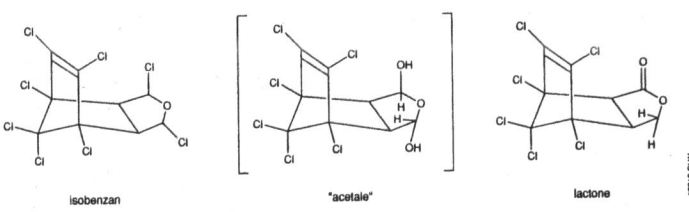

Fig. 1. Isobenzan, "acetale", and lactone.

a metabolite more hydrophilic than that produced by microorganisms. This metabolite consists of at least three components. The hydrolytic product of one of these components was identified as isobenzan lactone (Korte, 1963, 1967; Korte & Stiasni, 1964).

6.3.3 Microorganisms

Isobenzan labelled with ^{14}C in the hexachloropentane ring or at the 1,3 position is metabolized by the fungi *Aspergillus niger*, *Aspergillus flavus*, *Penicillium chrysogenum*, and *Penicillium notatum* to isobenzan lactone, the same metabolite as found in animal metabolism studies (Korte, 1963; Korte & Stiasni, 1964).

6.4 Elimination and excretion in expired air, faeces, and urine

6.4.1 Oral administration

In a study by Korte (1963), ten rabbits received in their diet 2 mg ^{14}C-isobenzan, diluted with non-radioactive isobenzan, every 2 days to a total amount of 25-30 mg per rabbit. After 3 months, about 50% of the total radioactivity administered had been excreted, mainly in the urine. On the other hand, rats excreted most of the radioactivity via bile into the gastrointestinal tract and excreted these products with the faeces. No unchanged isobenzan was excreted, only hydrophilic metabolites.

6.4.2 Parenteral administration

When Carworth Farm rats received daily intraperitoneal injections of isobenzan (98% purity) of 0.25, 1, or 2 mg/kg body weight 5 days per week for 2 weeks (section 7.2.3), they excreted less than 1% of the daily dose as unchanged isobenzan in the faeces (Brown et al., 1962).

In a study by Kaul et al. (1970), male and female rats received a single intravenous injection of 15 µg ^{14}C-isobenzan/kg body weight. The male rats excreted 1% of the applied radioactivity in the urine and 12% in the faeces within 48 h, while the females excreted 5% and 11%, respectively.

After having been administered intravenously to rats with cannulated bile ducts, ^{14}C-isobenzan was excreted as hydrophilic metabolites in the bile (Korte, 1963, 1967).

Male rabbits given an intravenous injection of ^{14}C-isobenzan (241 µg/kg body weight) excreted 12% in the urine and 1% in the faeces within 96 h (Kaul et al., 1970).

6.5 Retention and turnover

The absorption of isobenzan into the body is determined by measuring the insecticide in the blood. No human studies exist relating the concentration of isobenzan in the blood at the state of equilibrium to the total daily intake or relating the concentration of isobenzan in the blood to that in the tissues. However, in experimental animals, such relationships have been determined. Thus, in human beings, measurement of the blood concentration of the insecticide at the state of equilibrium is assumed to reflect total absorption by all routes (skin, pulmonary, and oral exposure) as well as the storage level in adipose tissue, thereby providing a measure of the total body burden of isobenzan.

From human data, it is estimated that the biological half-life of isobenzan in blood is of the order of 2.8 years (Jager, 1970) (section 8.2).

7. EFFECTS ON LABORATORY MAMMALS AND IN VITRO TEST SYSTEMS

7.1 Single exposure

7.1.1 Oral administration

In rats, the first signs of toxicity were evident approximately 1 h after the administration of a lethal dose and consisted of lethargy followed by muscular twitching, laboured breathing, and, finally, general convulsions. The majority of deaths occurred within the first 20 h after administration. No specific changes were observed in the organs of fatally intoxicated animals. Signs of intoxication were similar in mice, rats, guinea-pigs, cats, dogs, and chickens. Surviving animals recovered completely (Brown et al., 1962; Worden, 1969).

Oral LD_{50} values for the various animal species range from 1.6 to 10 mg/kg and are summarized in Table 5.

Table 5. Oral LD_{50} values for technical isobenzan

Species	Vehicle	LD_{50} (mg/kg body weight)	Reference
Mouse	arachis oil	10[a,b]	Worden (1969)
Mouse	corn oil	12.5	Spynu (1964)
Rat	corn oil	4.8	Howard et al. (1957)
Rat	corn oil	14.4	Spynu (1964)
Rat	carboxymethyl cellulose	5.4	Stevenson (1964)
Rat	dimethylsulfoxide	7.2	Stevenson (1964)
Rat	arachis oil	10[b]	Worden (1969)
Rat	unknown	8.0	Layton et al. (1987)
Guinea-pig	arachis oil	2.5[a,b]	Worden (1969)
Golden hamster	arachis oil	20[b]	Worden (1969)
Dog	unknown	1.6	Stevenson (1964)

[a] Average of males and females.
[b] Isobenzan 99.5%.

7.1.2 Dermal administration

Signs of intoxication are the same as those described for acute oral intoxication but they develop more slowly (Brown et al., 1962). The LD_{50} values are summarized in Table 6.

Table 6. Dermal LD_{50} values for technical isobenzan

Species	Vehicle	LD_{50} (mg/kg body weight)	Reference
Rat	arachis oil	occluded, 4 non-occluded, 10	Zavon (1961)
Rat	corn oil	non-occluded, 8.5	Spynu (1964)
Rat	crystalline form	occluded, 60 (approximately)	Stevenson (1964)

7.1.3 Parenteral administration

The acute toxicity of isobenzan administered parenterally is similar to that following oral administration (Table 7). The signs of intoxication are similar to those observed after acute oral toxicity but develop more rapidly, starting less than 1 h after the injection (Brown et al., 1962; Worden, 1969).

Table 7. Parenteral LD_{50} values for technical isobenzan

Route	Species	Vehicle	LD_{50} (mg/kg body weight)	Reference
Intraperitoneal	mouse	xylene emulsion	8.2	Stevenson (1964)
Intraperitoneal	mouse	methoxytriglycol	6.0	Cole & Casida (1986)
Intraperitoneal	rat	dimethylsulfoxide	3.6	Stevenson (1964)
Subcutaneous	rat, mouse	arachis oil	6-10	Worden (1969)
Intravenous	rat	unknown	1.7	Zavon (1961)

7.1.4 Formulated material

A 50% wettable powder formulation and a 15% emulsifiable concentrate (in mixed petroleum xylenes) were tested for their acute oral toxicity to rats, mice, rabbits, hamsters, cats, and dogs. The LD_{50} values, when expressed as active material, were comparable with those of isobenzan itself (Stevenson, 1964; Worden, 1969). The dermal LD_{50} value for the 15% emulsifiable concentrate was 25-35 mg isobenzan/kg body weight for Hooded-Lister rats and 6 mg isobenzan/kg body weight for New Zealand white rabbits, whereas in the case of the 50% wettable powder the LD_{50} was 41 mg isobenzan/kg body weight for rabbits (Stevenson, 1964). Rabbits exposed dermally to the 15% emulsifiable concentrate formulation behaved differently to rats similarly exposed. The rabbits generally lost weight due to anorexia and a failure to drink, and they would then convulse, even as much as 3 weeks after the exposure. However, if feeding and drinking were resumed quickly, the rabbits did not convulse (Brown, 1963, 1964).

7.1.5 Metabolites

The acute oral and intravenous toxicities of the metabolite isobenzan lactone for mice were 30 times lower than those of isobenzan. The oral and intravenous LD_{50} values were 306 mg/kg body weight and > 100 mg/kg body weight, respectively (Korte, 1967).

7.2 Short-term exposure

The short-term, long-term, and reproduction studies that were used for establishing a no-observed-effect level are summarized in Table 8.

7.2.1 Oral administration

7.2.1.1 Mouse

In a study by Brown et al. (1962), groups of five male and five female Carworth Farm No. 1 mice were fed diets containing isobenzan (98%) at levels of 1, 2, 3, 4, or 5 mg/kg for up to 3 weeks. No mortality was observed at 1 mg/kg, but at the higher concentrations the mortality was dose related, reaching 100% at 5 mg/kg diet.

Table 8. Short- and long-term oral exposure to isobenzan

Animal (strain)	Exposure period	NOAEL[a] (mg/kg diet)	LOAEL[a] (mg/kg diet)	References
Rat (Sprague-Dawley)	30 days	2.5 (0.12)	12.5 (0.62): irritability, decreased body weight gain, histopathology changes in heart	Howard et al. (1957)
Dog (Beagle)	2 years	(0.08)	(0.125): convulsion, mortality	Brown & Richardson (1964)
Dog (Scottish terrier)	2 years	(0.025)	(0.1): decreased body weight gain, increased liver weight	Worden (1969)
Rat (Hooded-Lister)	2 years	5 (0.25)	17.5 (0.87): convulsions	Worden (1969)
Reproduction study				
Rat (Carworth Farm)	one generation (2 litters)	0.1 (0.005) (pups) 1.0 (0.05) (parents)	1 (0.05): decreased survival of pups 5 (0.25): convulsions	Chambers (1962a,b)

[a] Figures in parentheses are values for exposure concentration in mg/kg body weight.

7.2.1.2 Rat

Groups of eight male and eight female Carworth Farm rats were intubated with isobenzan (98%) in dimethylsulfoxide (0.25, 1, or 2.5 mg/kg body weight per day) 5 days/week for 2 weeks. All rats dosed with 2.5 mg/kg body weight died within 5 days. All the females and two of the males dosed with 1 mg/kg body weight died after 5-7 doses, whereas only one female dosed with 0.25 mg/kg body weight died after five doses. Weight loss preceded the death of the animals at the highest dose, this being the result of reduced food intake. No gross or microscopic changes were found in the rats dying from intoxication or in the survivors sacrificed 14 days after the last treatment (no details were reported concerning the parameters studied) (Brown et al., 1962).

In a study by Howard et al. (1957), groups of 10 male and 10 female Sprague-Dawley rats were fed diets containing 0, 2.5, 12.5, or 25 mg isobenzan/kg diet for 30 days. One female in the highest-dose group died. Some of the rats fed with levels of 12.5 or 25 mg/kg were nervous and irritable, and the reduced body weight gain in both these groups correlated with diminished food consumption. At autopsy, there were some areas of necrosis of heart cells and haemorrhages in the heart muscle of animals fed with levels of 12.5 or 25 mg/kg diet.

In a study by Worden (1969), groups of five male and five female Hooded-Lister rats were fed diets containing isobenzan (99.5%) (25, 35, 50, or 100 mg/kg diet) as a 15% emulsifiable concentrate (in mixed petroleum xylenes). After 37 days on the test diets, half of the surviving animals of each group were transferred to a control diet, while the remainder continued on the test diets for a further 42 days. During the first period, all rats fed with 100 mg/kg diet died except for one male. One male and two females fed with 50 mg/kg diet died as did three females fed with 35 mg/kg diet. There were no further deaths among the rats after dosing was discontinued. During the second period of feeding with the test diet, one female fed at the lowest level died. In one rat only, a female fed with 50 mg/kg, the classical signs of organochlorine intoxication were seen in the liver. These have been described by Hodge et al. (1967) as "enlarged centrolobular hepatic cells with cytoplasmic oxyphilia and somewhat increased and peripheral migration of the basophilic granules".

7.2.1.3 Dog

Pairs of Beagle hounds (one male and one female) were given daily oral doses of 0, 0.08, 0.125, or 0.2 mg isobenzan (98%)/kg body weight in olive oil in gelatin capsules for 2 years. The dogs given the two highest doses had several convulsive episodes during the course of the study. When a dog exhibited a convulsion, dosing was discontinued for 8 weeks. The male dog dosed with 0.125 mg/kg died one week after a third convulsive episode, which followed a sudden fall in body weight. No signs of intoxication were observed in the dogs dosed with 0.08 mg/kg body weight. During this study, blood isobenzan concentrations were measured regularly, in particular at the time of convulsions. Concentrations in muscle tissue were determined 3 days after the convulsion, and the results are given in Table 9. The blood concentrations in the dogs receiving 0.08 mg/kg body weight for 2 years without convulsions indicated that a plateau was reached after a relatively short exposure. The mean concentration was approximately 0.02 mg isobenzan/litre and the maximum concentration 0.04-0.05 mg/litre. The two highest doses caused convulsions (Brown & Richardson, 1964).

Table 9. Concentration of isobenzan in the blood and muscle of dogs

Dose (mg/kg body weight)	Sex	Number of convulsions	Blood concentration at time of convulsion (mg/litre)	Muscle tissue (mg/kg wet weight)
0.08	male	none	0.04 (maximum concentration)	
	female	none	0.05 (maximum concentration)	
0.125	male	first two third (death)	0.06 0.11	16
	female	4	0.03-0.06	0.18
0.2	male	9	0.02-0.11	0.36
	female	6	0.07-0.08	0.68

Groups of three male and three female Scottish terriers (2.5-9 kg body weight) received daily gavage doses of isobenzan (0, 0.025, or 0.1 mg/kg body weight) as 15% emulsifiable concentrate (in mixed petroleum xylenes) for 2 years. No deaths and no signs of intoxication resulted from the isobenzan administration. Body weight gain, urinalysis, and haematological and clinical chemistry values for the dogs fed with 0.025 mg/kg body weight were comparable with those of the control animals. At a dose level of 0.1 mg/kg body weight, a decrease in body weight gain, a slight increase in serum alkaline phosphatase values during the second year, and an increase in liver weight were noted. No evidence of histopathological lesions attributable to isobenzan was found at either treatment level. The no-observed-effect level resulting from this study was 0.025 mg/kg body weight (Worden, 1969). The distribution of isobenzan in the tissues examined is summarized in section 6.2.2.

7.2.2 Dermal administration

When groups of five female albino rabbits were given daily applications of isobenzan in corn oil (0, 5, 10, 20, 30, or 40 mg per rabbit) to the shaven skin for 3 weeks, mortality was high at all dose levels, reaching 100% after 2 weeks for rabbits given doses of 30 or 40 mg. Histopathological examination revealed necrosis of the heart muscle, non-dose-related lesions of the liver, and degenerative changes in cells of the central nervous system in a few animals (Howard et al., 1957).

7.2.3 Intraperitoneal administration

Groups of five male and five female Carworth Farm rats were injected intraperitoneally with isobenzan (98%) in dimethyl-sulfoxide (0.25, 1, or 2 mg/kg body weight per day) 5 days/week for 2 weeks. All rats given the lowest dose survived, but two rats of each sex given 1 mg/kg and five males and four females given 2 mg/kg died after 5-10 doses. No gross or microscopic lesions were found in fatally intoxicated rats or in the survivors killed 7-14 days after the last treatment (no details concerning parameters studied were reported) (Brown et al., 1962).

7.3 Long-term exposure

7.3.1 Rat

Groups of 25 male and 25 female Hooded-Lister rats were fed, at dietary concentrations of 5, 17.5, or 30 mg/kg (equivalent to 0.25, 0.875, or 1.5 mg/kg body weight), isobenzan as a 15% emulsifiable concentrate (in mixed petroleum xylenes) for 2 years.

Three control groups, each consisting of 25 male and 25 female rats, were used. Additional groups of rats, fed at the same dose levels and accompanied by separate control groups, were used for liver and kidney function tests after 20, 66, and 104 weeks. Five females fed at the highest dose level died during the first 3 weeks of the study. Signs of intoxication (such as ruffled coat, lethargy, muscular twitches, and mild to violent convulsions) were observed in animals given 17.5 or 30 mg/kg diet, mainly during the first few weeks. There were no adverse effects on body weight gain, food conversion ratios, haematological parameters, serum alkaline phosphatase, serum glutamic-pyruvic transaminase, total serum protein, or albumin/globulin ratios. Absolute liver weight was increased in the animals given the highest dose level. Gross and microscopic examinations did not reveal any compound-related changes, with the possible exception of thyroid hyperplasia recorded in four males and six females at a level of 30 mg/kg diet. The liver function test (bromsulfophthalein) and kidney function test (phenol red) showed no deviations from control values. No significant increase in the number and type of tumours was found. The no-observed-effect level for toxicological effects was 5 mg isobenzan/kg diet (equivalent to 0.25 mg/kg body weight) for 2 years (Worden, 1969).

7.4 Skin irritation

In a study by Worden (1969), four male guinea-pigs received a single application (2 mg/kg body weight) of isobenzan (99.5%) as a 0.2% w/v solution in arachis oil to the shaved skin. The material was not removed from the skin. The animals were kept under observation for 21 days, but no irritation was observed.

Two male and two female rabbits were given 12 successive daily applications (0.5 mg/kg body weight) of isobenzan (99.5%) and six female rats received 30 successive daily applications (0.3 mg/kg body weight) of isobenzan as a 0.2% w/v solution in arachis oil to the shaved skin. The material was left on the skin and the observation period was 21 days after the last application. No irritation was observed (Worden, 1969).

7.5 Reproductive toxicity, embryotoxicity, and teratogenicity

No studies on the potential teratogenicity of isobenzan have been reported.

7.5.1 Mouse

In a range-finding test, groups of 25 male and 25 female BALB/C mice were fed diets containing 0, 1, 2.5, 5, or 10 mg isobenzan (94%)/kg. The mice in the 5- and 10-mg/kg dose groups all died within 64 and 24 days, respectively. Only 20% of those in the 2.5-mg/kg group survived for 120 days. The 1 mg/kg group survived and reproduced normally (no further data were reported). In the main study, groups of 108 mice of each sex of Swiss strain BALB/C were fed control diet and 106 mice of each sex were fed 1 mg isobenzan/kg diet for 30 days, after which they were randomly paired and continued on the same diet for 90 days. The number of litters produced, litter size, sex ratio, and mortality were recorded in this one-generation reproduction study. There were no statistically significant differences between the control and isobenzan-treated animals for any of the parameters measured (Ware & Good, 1967).

7.5.2 Rat

A one-generation, 2-litter reproduction study was carried out with groups of 20 male and 20 female weanling Carworth Farm rats that were fed diets containing isobenzan at levels of 0, 0.1, 1, 5, or 10 mg/kg for 100 days and then mated. Convulsions were seen during the mating period and pregnancy in females fed 10 mg/kg, and during the lactation period in one female fed 5 mg/kg. Pups of the second mating from both these treatment groups were also seen to convulse. Mean litter size and survival of pups were markedly reduced in the 10-mg/kg group and, to a lesser extent, in the 5-mg/kg group. No clinical signs were observed in the 1-mg/kg group. At this dose level, the mean litter size was comparable with controls, but survival of the pups at 21 days was decreased. No effects attributable to isobenzan were found in the 0.1-mg/kg group (Chambers, 1962a,b).

7.5.3 Dog

During a 2-year study (section 7.2.1.3), three litters were born to a female Beagle hound dosed daily with 0.08 mg isobenzan/kg body weight five days per week. A male Beagle dog, dosed at the same level, was sire for several of the litters. The first litter consisted of one male and one female, both normal, and one still-born male. Fifteen days after birth, the female pup began to convulse, having only fed on the mother's milk (which contained 0.7 mg isobenzan/litre) and at 17 days the pup was sacrificed.

Concentrations of isobenzan in tissues are given in section 6.2.2. Two further litters of pups were born to the original dam (two male pups in the first litter and two pups of each sex in the second). These animals all appeared normal and healthy and showed no ill effects from the ingestion of maternal milk. One litter of pups, one male and one female, was born to a female Beagle dog fed 0.125 mg/kg body weight per day for two years. These pups did not exhibit any signs of intoxication and were killed when 26 days old. Autopsy did not reveal any structural changes. It did not appear that isobenzan interfered with either the male or female reproduction function (Brown & Richardson, 1964).

7.6 Mutagenicity and related end-points

No information on mutagenicity is available.

7.7 Carcinogenicity

No *adequate* carcinogenicity studies have been reported.

7.7.1 Mouse

Groups of 18 male and 18 female mice of two hybrid strains (the F_1 hybrids C57Bl/6 x C3H/Anf and C57Bl/6 x AKR) were given the maximum tolerated dose of isobenzan in 0.5% gelatin (0.215 mg/kg body weight) daily from 7 to 28 days of age by stomach tube. Thereafter the isobenzan was mixed in the diet to a concentration of 0.646 mg/kg, and the mice were killed at 18 months of age. No significant increase in tumour incidence was found (Innes et al., 1969).

7.7.2 Rat

In a long-term feeding study on rats (section 7.4.1), no evidence of carcinogenicity was found as a result of feeding diets containing up to 30 mg isobenzan/kg for 2 years (Worden, 1969).

7.8 Special studies

7.8.1 Biochemical studies

Mehrotra et al. (1982) studied the comparative effects of cyclodiene compounds on different ATPase activities in beef and rat brain synaptosomal fractions *in vitro*. Isobenzan significantly inhibited Na^+-K^+-ATPase in rat brain synaptosomes. A dose-related response was observed at up to 80 µmol/litre, but no increase in inhibition was observed with a further increase in the concentration of the compound. Oligomycin-sensitive Mg^{2+}-ATPase in rat brain synaptosomes was significantly inhibited by isobenzan, a maximum of 64% inhibition occurring at 120 µmol/litre. In addition, the oligomycin-insensitive Mg^{2+}-ATPase in rat brain synaptosomes was inhibited, and the inhibition was concentration dependent. Isobenzan did not have any effect on K^+-stimulated p-nitrophenylphosphatase, an enzyme which is known to represent the dephosphorylation step in the overall reaction of the Na^+-K^+-ATPase. Oligomycin-sensitive Mg^{2+}-ATPase in beef heart mitochondria was significantly inhibited.

Isobenzan did not affect the activity of adenylate cyclase or phosphodiesterase in Sprague-Dawley rat brain synaptosomes *in vitro* at concentrations of up to 200 µmol/litre (Kodavanti et al., 1988).

Several studies into the effect of isobenzan on the transfer of ammonia in brain have indicated that isobenzan acts by increasing brain ammonia levels before and during convulsions. Glutamic acid, glutamine, and alpha-ketoglutaric acid, which are utilized in an ammonia-binding mechanism, become overwhelmed, resulting in free ammonia accumulating in the cerebral tissues (Hathway & Mallinson, 1964; Hathway, 1965; Hathway et al., 1965).

7.8.2 Neurotoxicity

In vitro studies using fresh rat brain synaptic membranes showed isobenzan to be a potent inhibitor of the binding of the convulsant *tert*-butylbicyclophosphorothionate (TBPS) to brain-specific sites, thereby indicating an action at the gamma-aminobutyric acid (GABA)-regulated chloride channel. Metabolic activation by rat liver microsomes did not enhance the potency for inhibition. This inhibition indicates that isobenzan binds to the same site as TBPS, suggesting that isobenzan acts in a manner similar to non-competitive GABA-A antagonists and providing a basis for its convulsant action in mammals (Lawrence & Casida, 1984).

Bloomquist et al. (1986) produced a concentration-dependent inhibition of ^{36}Cl uptake into mouse brain vesicles by adding isobenzan to mouse brain homogenate. The inhibitory activity was confined to that portion of ^{36}Cl uptake that was GABA dependent.

The insecticide concentration producing 50% inhibition (I_{50}) of ^{36}Cl uptake was 2.0 (0.83 to 5.1) µmol/litre, and the inhibitory potency (I_{50}) value for ^{35}S-TBPS binding in rat brain synaptosomes was 0.30 µmol/litre (Lawrence & Casida, 1984).

Cole & Casida (1986) confirmed in a study with male Swiss-Webster mice administered isobenzan intraperitoneally that a correlation also exist *in vivo* between binding to mouse brain GABA receptors and convulsive activity. The inhibitory potency (IC_{50}) for *in vitro* TBPS binding to mouse brain synaptosomes is 0.03 µmol/litre. It was shown that the inhibitory potencies of cyclodienes, including isobenzan, parallel their acute oral toxicities. Isobenzan was slightly more potent than endrin and produced virtually complete inhibition of GABA-dependent chloride uptake at 30 µmol/litre. There was a significant linear correlation between the ^{36}Cl flux and ^{35}S-TBPS-binding assays.

7.8.3 Pharmacological studies

Pharmacological studies on the function of organ systems in various animal species (such as rats, guinea-pigs, rabbits, cats, and frogs) after the administration of isobenzan by different routes showed that the only significant effect was a disturbance of the central nervous system associated with convulsions. This effect was due to stimulation of the higher brain centres at the level of the medulla and above. Changes in respiratory rate, heart rate, and salivary secretion were probably mediated by the central nervous system as a secondary effect of central nervous stimulation. Barbiturates were found to control these convulsions. The stimulation of brain activity was reflected in the occurrence of electroencephalographic changes in the pre-convulsive stage and during the convulsive episodes. This corresponds to the situation in cases of human intoxication by occupational exposure to cyclodiene insecticides as described by Hoogendam et al. (1962, 1965) and Chambers (1962c).

Ibrahim (1964) showed that isobenzan injected intraperitoneally at a toxic dose (7 mg/kg body weight) into male Wistar rats produced a higher tension of contraction in the gastrocnemius muscle at lower frequencies of stimulation than in controls. The maximum tetanic tension was also attained at a lower frequency. An increase in the duration of the "active state" of the muscle was considered to be the most like explanation.

8. EFFECTS ON HUMANS

8.1 General population exposure

No poisoning incidents or untoward effects of long-term exposure of the general population have been reported.

8.2 Occupational exposure

Isobenzan was initially manufactured and handled in the Netherlands between 1958 and 1965. Aldrin, dieldrin, and endrin were also produced in the same manufacturing plant and, consequently, in many cases the exposure was mixed. Routine medical examination of 233 workers, who were exposed for more than 4 years and who followed normal procedures during that period, did not reveal any abnormalities in EEG, clinical chemistry or haematological parameters, or liver microsomal enzyme induction (Jager, 1970; Versteeg & Jager, 1973). The mean isobenzan concentration in the blood of 20 operators after cessation of exposure decreased from 22 µg/litre in 1965 to 7 µg/litre in 1969. The biological half-life of isobenzan in the blood (at the state of equilibrium of isobenzan in body tissues) was estimated to be of the order of 2.8 years (Jager, 1970).

In the 7 years of isobenzan production, 15 cases of clinical intoxication, including eight cases with convulsions, were reported. The mean concentration of isobenzan in the blood of nine workers at the time of intoxication was 23 µg/litre, the range being 17-30 µg/litre. Although these workers recovered fully, it took longer than with the related cyclodiene insecticides. In three cases, certain typical complaints, such as headache, dizziness, drowsiness, and irritability, persisted for 6 months, and the return to normal of the modified EEG pattern sometimes took more than a year. In one case of acute over-exposure, without signs of intoxication, the blood isobenzan concentration decreased from 8 µg/litre to less than 2 µg/litre within 3 days (Jager, 1970).

The data from plant workers indicated a threshold level of isobenzan in blood below which no signs or symptoms of intoxication occur. This level was found to be 15 µg/litre (Jager, 1970).

Ribbens (1985) carried out a mortality study on the abovementioned industrial workers exposed to aldrin, dieldrin, endrin, and isobenzan. Vital status and cause of death were assessed for 232 of the total population of more than 1000 workers. This group was selected for follow-up on account of the high degree of exposure in the initial years of manufacturing and formulation and the long exposure (mean 11 years) and observation (mean 24 years) periods. Total observed mortality was 25 as opposed to 38 expected on the basis of death statistics for the male Dutch population. Of the nine cancer deaths, three were caused by lung cancer, while the remaining six were each of a different nature. The author concluded that although exposures in this group were high and exposure as well as observation periods long, this study did not reveal any indication of a specific carcinogenic activity of these pesticides.

9. EFFECTS ON OTHER ORGANISMS IN THE LABORATORY AND FIELD

9.1 Microorganisms

In laboratory studies, sandy loam soil was treated with 250 or 2500 mg isobenzan/kg (concentrations that exceeded the recommended rates). At both concentrations, the carbon dioxide production was inhibited to almost the same extent (21 and 24%, respectively) during a 30-day test period. The addition of glucose to the soil reduced the inhibitory effect to 5 and 4%, respectively. Isobenzan at 250 mg/kg did not influence nitrification in the soil up to 18 days after treatment (Bartha et al., 1967).

Screening studies on microorganisms in pure culture were carried out on nutrient agar plates with isobenzan either incorporated in a uniformly emulsified form (1000 mg/kg) or as a thin surface film (1 mg/cm^2). The growth of the gram-positive *Bacillus megaterium* was inhibited, but not that of various gram-negative organisms such as several *Pseudomonas* strains, *Escherichia coli*, *Klebsiella aerogenes* W5, or *Achromobacter butyri* (Trudgill & Widdus, 1970).

9.2 Aquatic organisms

Groups of five adult Harlequin fish *(Rasbora heteromorpha)* were exposed for 2 h at a temperature of 20 °C to water (pH 7.2) containing isobenzan (99%), dissolved in DMSO, at a concentration of 0.01, 0.1, or 1 mg/litre. The fish were then transferred to clean water and observed for an additional 48 h. The treatment with 1 mg/litre caused disorientation and the fish became excited by external stimuli, lost the ability to swim, and, finally, all died within 1 h. In some cases, they appeared to convulse. Isobenzan at 0.1 mg/litre caused similar symptoms; within 2 h of exposure, all five fish died. No fish died at 0.01 mg/litre, but slight changes in swimming behaviour were observed (Brown et al., 1962). When guppies *(Poecilia reticulata)* were tested in the same way, the symptoms of intoxication and susceptibility were similar to those in Harlequin fish, but the guppies were slower to react (Brown et al., 1962).

Data on the acute toxicity of isobenzan for aquatic organisms in flow-through tests are given in Table 10.

Table 10. Acute toxicity of isobenzan (technical grade, 94%) for aquatic organisms

Organism	Developmental stage	Temperature (°C)	Parameter	Concentration (μg/litre)	Reference
Brown shrimp (*Penaeus aztecus*)	juvenile	17	48-h EC$_{50}$	0.034[a]	US EPA (1987)
Eastern oyster (*Crassostrea virginica*)	juvenile	18	96-h EC$_{50}$	32[b]	US EPA (1987)
Sheepshead minnow (*Cyprinodon variegatus*)	juvenile	17	48-h LC$_{50}$	2.0[a]	US EPA (1987)
Spot (*Leiostomus xanthurus*)	juvenile	13	48-h LC$_{50}$	0.32[c]	US EPA (1987)

[a] Salinity 30 ng/litre.
[b] Salinity 33 ng/litre.
[c] Salinity 22 ng/litre.

9.3 Terrestrial organisms

9.3.1 Soil invertebrates

In laboratory studies, plain-field sand was treated once with 0.05 mg isobenzan/kg and stored at 13 or 24 °C. The springtail *(Folsomia candida)* was used for bioassays lasting up to 16 weeks. The biological activity of isobenzan persisted slightly longer at the higher temperature, killing 100% of the insects after 16 weeks (Thompson, 1973).

9.3.2 Birds

9.3.2.1 Acute toxicity

Isobenzan (> 99%) is highly toxic to birds when administered as a single oral dose (Table 11). LD$_{50}$ values range from 1-10 mg/kg.

9.3.2.2 Short-term toxicity

When groups of five male and five female Japanese quail *(Coturnix coturnix japonica)* were fed diets containing 2 or 10 mg isobenzan/kg, the mean survival time in the high-dose group was 6.9 days (range, 2-20 days). The residues in the liver and brain averaged 3.4 mg/kg and 1.4 mg/kg, respectively. In the low-dose group, the mean survival time was 45.9 days (range, 19-65 days) and the average residues in liver and brain were 6 mg/kg and 1.6 mg/kg, respectively. The concentration of isobenzan in the liver of birds fed 2 mg/kg was significantly higher than that in the high-dose group, but the concentration in the brain showed no difference (Koeman, 1971).

Table 11. Oral LD_{50} values of isobenzan for birds

Species	LD_{50} (mg/kg body weight)	Reference
Mallard duck (female) (*Anas platyrhynchos*)	4.15 (2.47-6.97)	Hudson et al. (1984)
Coturnix quail (female) (*Coturnix coturnix*)	4.2	Schafer & Brunton (1979)
Grackle (*Quiscalus quiscula*)	1.3	Schafer & Brunton (1979)
Pigeon (*Columba livia*)	10	Schafer & Brunton (1979)
Red-winged blackbird (male) (*Agelaius phoeniceus*)	3.2	Schafer & Brunton (1979)
Sparrow (*Passer domesticus*)	1	Schafer & Brunton (1979)
Starling (*Sturnus vulgaris*)	2.4	Schafer & Brunton (1979)

When groups of 20 Rhode Island Red laying hens were fed isobenzan (15% emulsifiable concentrate) at levels of 0.1, 0.25, 0.75, or 1 mg/kg diet for 14 weeks, no effects were seen on food consumption, egg production, egg weight, or egg fertility (Verma et al., 1967).

9.4 Population and ecosystem effects

9.4.1 Soil microorganisms

In a sugar cane field in India, Srivastava (1966) studied the effect of isobenzan (1 kg/ha) on nitrification of ammonium sulfate in the soil. The insecticide-treated soil contained higher amounts of total inorganic nitrogen and ammonium nitrogen (80% increase) up to 60 days after treatment than did untreated soil samples, indicating impaired nitrification.

9.4.2 Soil invertebrates

In a study by Kelsey & Arlidge (1968), five sandy loam plots of pasture in New Zealand were treated with Telodrin (15% emulsifiable concentrate) at a rate of 2 kg isobenzan/ha in June 1962. The populations of all recorded groups (grass grub, porina, Collembola, Diptera, Hemiptera, Coleoptera, mites, and earthworms), except nematodes, were drastically reduced. There was no recovery in the populations of any of the affected groups during the period up to October 1965. In silt loam plots treated with isobenzan granules (1 kg/ha) in April 1964, the populations of Coleoptera, Collembola, Diptera, mites, and earthworms were all reduced, but to a lesser extent than in the test using 2 kg/ha. However, grass grub and Hemiptera were not significantly affected, and nematode numbers were elevated 2 years after the treatment. Studies on root development showed that 90% of roots with root hairs were located within a mat of plant debris above the soil, whereas in controls 99% were located in the soil. Plant growth was retarded. The moisture content of the treated plots was significantly less than that of control plots, indicating that the capacity of soil to absorb and retain water had been reduced.

When loose sandy soil in New Zealand was treated with 2.25 kg isobenzan/ha as 5% granules, the population reduction, 1-18 weeks after treatment, was 90-100% for larval Coleoptera and Lepidoptera and 75% for Diptera and earthworms. The number of surface arthropods, 5-15 days after treatment, was reduced by 45%. Six months after treatment, little effect was found on nematodes (13% reduction), bacteria (18% reduction), and fungi (7% increase) (Moeed, 1975).

REFERENCES

ANON (1974) Aldrin, dieldrin, and endrin. Determination of residues of organochlorine insecticides in crops, soils, and animal products, Sittingbourne, Shell Research (Residue Analytical Method WAMS 60-1).

BARTHA, R., LANZILOTTA, R.P., & PRAMER, D. (1967) Stability and effects of some pesticides in soil. Appl. Microbiol., 15(1): 67-75.

BAUER, U. (1972) [Behaviour of a series of plant-protecting agents during the treatment of groundwater by slow sand filtration.] Schriftenr. Ver. Wasser-Boden-Lufthyg. (Berlin-Dahlem), 37: 91-102 (in German).

BIEHL, M.L. & BUCK, H.B. (1987) Chemical contaminants: their metabolism and their residues. J. Food Prot., 50(12): 1058-1073.

BISHOP, J.L. & HUBER, J.T. (1964) Secretion of Telodrin in the milk of cows fed varying levels of Telodrin. J. dairy Sci., 47: 552-554.

BLOOMQUIST, J.R., ADAMS, P.M., & SÖDERLAND, D.M. (1986) Inhibition of gamma-aminobutyric acid stimulated chloride flux in mouse brain vesicles by polychlorocycloalkane and pyrethroid insecticides. Neurotoxicology, 7(3): 11-20.

BOWMAN, M.C., SCHECHTER, M.S., & CARTER, R.L. (1965) Behavior of chlorinated insecticides in a broad spectrum of soil types. J. agric. food Chem., 13: 360-365.

BROWN, V.K.H. (1963) Agricultural chemicals: the relative percutaneous toxicities of Nitrophoska fertiliser granules impregnated with aldrin and Telodrin, Sittingbourne, Shell Research (Technical Memorandum TOX 10/63).

BROWN, V.K.H. (1964) Some effects of percutaneously absorbed Telodrin in rabbits, Sittingbourne, Shell Research (Report No. PPR TL/2/64).

BROWN, V.K.H. & RICHARDSON, A. (1964) Chronic oral exposure of beagle hounds to Telodrin and dieldrin: report on the first two years, Sittingbourne, Shell Research (Report No. PPR TL/1/64).

BROWN, V.K.H., CHAMBERS, P.L., HUNTER, C.G., & STEVENSON, D.E. (1962) The toxicity of Telodrin for vertebrates, Sittingbourne, Shell Research (Report No. R(T)-2-62).

BUICK, A.R. (1964) Telodrin residues on tobacco from Australia, Sittingbourne, Shell International Chemical Company, Ltd (Technical Memorandum 132/64)

BUICK, A.R. (1965) Telodrin residues in potatoes from India, Sittingbourne, Shell International Chemical Company, Ltd (Technical Memorandum 25/65).

BUICK, A.R. & COLE, E.R. (1965) Telodrin residues in sweet potatoes from South Africa, Sittingbourne, Shell International Chemical Company, Ltd (Technical Memorandum 25/65).

BULL, M.S. & MARLOW, R.G. (1967) Insecticide residues in diet samples from Nicaragua, Sittingbourne, Shell International Chemical Company, Ltd (Technical Service Note 85/67).

References

BULL, M.S. & RAMSDEN, D.P. (1967) Residues of organochlorine insecticides in samples from Venezuela, Sittingbourne, Shell International Chemical Company, Ltd (Technical Service Note 86/67).

CHAMBERS, P.L. (1962a) Agricultural chemicals: the effect of Telodrin on reproduction in the rat when fed at various levels in the diet. Report No. 3, Sittingbourne, Shell International Chemical Company, Ltd (Technical Memorandum TOX 24/62).

CHAMBERS, P.L. (1962b) Agricultural chemicals: the effect of Telodrin on reproduction in the rat when fed at various levels in the diet. Report No. 4, Sittingbourne, Shell International Chemical Company, Ltd (Technical Memorandum TOX 33/62).

CHAMBERS, P.L. (1962c) The physiological and pharmacological effects of Telodrin, Sittingbourne, Shell Research (Report No. M(T)-4-62).

COLE, L.M. & CASIDA, J.E. (1986) Polychlorocycloalkane insecticide-induced convulsions in mice in relation to disruption of the GABA-regulated chloride ionophore. Life Sci., 39: 1855-1862.

CRABTREE, A.N. (1968) Concentration of chlorinated insecticides in the whole blood of the CAPSA plant in Venezuela, Sittingbourne, Shell Research (Report No. TLGR.0032.68).

DAVIES, J.M. (1966a) Chlorinated insecticide content of the blood of formulators in the CAPSA plant in Venezuela, Sittingbourne, Shell Research (Report No. IRR TL/14/66).

DAVIES, J.M. (1966b) Concentration of chlorinated insecticides in the whole blood of formulators of the CAPSA plant in Venezuela, Sittingbourne, Shell Research (Report No. IRR TL/37/66).

EDWARDS, C.A. (1965) Effects of pesticide residues on soil invertebrates and plants. In: Proceedings of the 5th Symposium of the British Ecological Society, Ecology and Industrial Society.

EICHELBERGER, J.W. & LICHTENBERG, J.J. (1971) Persistence of pesticides in river water. Environ. Sci. Technol., 5(6): 541-544.

ELGAR, K.E. (1965) Insecticide residues in samples of cottonseed from Mexico, Sittingbourne, Shell International Chemical Company, Ltd (Technical Memorandum 99/65).

ELGAR, K.E. (1966) Analysis of crops and soils for residues of the soil insecticides aldrin and Telodrin. J. Sci. Food Agric., 17: 541-545.

ELGAR, K.E. & HOLLAND, A.A. (1967) Residues of organochlorine insecticides in potatoes from Mexico, Sittingbourne, Shell International Chemical Company, Ltd (Technical Service Note 82/67).

HARDEE, D.D., GUTENMANN, W.H., KEENAN, G.I., GYRISCO, G.G., LISK, D.J., FOX, F.H., TRIMBERGER, G.W., & HOLLAND, R.F. (1964) Residues of heptachlor epoxide and Telodrin in milk from cows fed at parts per billion insecticide levels. J. econ. Entomol., 56(3): 404-407.

HATHWAY, D.E. (1965) The biochemistry of dieldrin and Telodrin. Arch. environ. Health, 11: 380-388.

HATHWAY, D.E. & MALLINSON, A. (1964) Chemical studies in relation to convulsive conditions: effect of Telodrin on the liberation and utilization of ammonia in rat brain. Biochem. J., 90: 51-60.

HATHWAY, D.E., MALLINSON, A., & AKINTONWA, D.A.A. (1965) Effects of dieldrin, picrotoxin, and Telodrin on the metabolism of ammonia in brain. Biochem. J., 94: 676-686.

HODGE, H.C., BOYCE, A.M., DEICHMANN, W.B., & KRAYBILL, H.F. (1967) Toxicology and no-effect levels of aldrin and dieldrin. Toxicol. appl. Pharmacol., 10(3): 613-637.

HOOGENDAM, I., VERSTEEG, J.P.J., & VLIEGER, M., DE (1962) Electroencephalograms in insecticide toxicity. Arch. environ. Health, 4: 86-94.

HOOGENDAM, I., VERSTEEG, J.P.J., & VLIEGER, M., DE (1965) Nine years toxicity control in insecticide plants. Arch. environ. Health, 10: 441-448.

HOWARD, J.A., BUXTON, J.A., ATER, F.B., OVERBECK, R.C., FOOTE, W.L., ROBINSON, R.F., & DAVIDSON, R.S. (1957) Final report on toxicology of BAS-4402 to the Shell Development Corporation, Columbus, Ohio, Battelle Memorial Institute.

HUDSON, R.H., TUCKER, R.K., & HAEGELE, M.A. (1984) Handbook of toxicity of pesticides to wildlife. 2nd ed., Washington, DC, US Department of the Interior, Fish and Wildlife Service (Resource Publication No. 153).

HUGHES, D.G. (1965) Insecticide residues in cottonseed oil, Sittingbourne, Shell International Chemical Company, Ltd (Technical Memorandum 23/65).

IBRAHIM, T.M. (1964) A toxicological study of the action of the insecticide dieldrin and related substances on the contraction of striated muscle in the rat, University of Utrecht (Thesis).

INNES, J.R.M., ULLAND, B.M., VALERIO, M.G., PETRUCELLI, L., FISHBEIN, L., HART, E.R., PALLOTTA, A.J., BATES, R.R., FALK, H.L., GART, J.J., KLEIN, M., MITCHELL, I., & PETERS, J. (1969) Bioassay of pesticides and industrial chemicals for tumorigenicity in mice: a preliminary note. J. Natl Cancer Inst., 42(6): 1101-1114.

JAGER, K.W. (1970) Aldrin, dieldrin, endrin, and Telodrin: an epidemiological and toxicological study of long-term occupational exposure, Amsterdam, London, New York, Elsevier Science Publishers.

JAPANESE ENVIRONMENTAL AGENCY (1975) Environmental survey report on chemical substances in FY 1974, Tokyo, Environmental Health Department, Planning and Coordination Bureau (Unpublished report).

KADOUM, A.M. (1968) Application of the rapid micro method of sample clean-up for gas chromatographic analysis of common organic pesticides in ground water, soil, plant and animal extracts. Bull. environ. Contam. Toxicol., 3(2): 65-70.

References

KAUL, R., KLEIN, W., & KORTE, F. (1970) [Contributions to ecological chemistry. XX. Distribution, elimination, and metabolism of Telodrin and heptachlor in rats and male rabbits, end-product of the metabolism of heptachlor in mammals.] Tetrahedron, 26: 331-337 (in German).

KELSEY, J.M. & ARLIDGE, E.Z. (1968) Effects of isobenzan on soil fauna and soil structure. N. Z. J. agric. Res., 11: 245-260.

KERDIJK, H.N. (1981) Groundwater pollution by heavy metals and pesticides from a dredge spoil dump. Stud. environ. Sci., 17: 279-286.

KODAVANTI, P.R.S., MEHROTRA, R.D., CHETTY, S.C., & DESAIAH, D. (1988) Effect of selected insecticides on rat brain synaptosomal adenylate cyclase and phosphodiesterase. J. Toxicol. environ. Health, 25: 207-215.

KOEMAN, J.H. (1971) [The occurrence and toxicological implications of some chlorinated hydrocarbons in the Dutch coastal area in the period from 1965 to 1970], University of Utrecht, pp. 30-31 (Thesis) (in Dutch).

KOEMAN, J.H., OSKAMP, A.A.G., VEEN, J., BROUWER, E., ROOTH, J., ZWART, P., VAN DE BROEK, E., & VAN GENDEREN, H. (1967) Insecticides as a factor in the mortality of the sandwich tern *(Sterna sandvicensis)*: a preliminary communication. Meded. Landbouwwet. Hogesch. Gent., 32: 841-854.

KOEMAN, J.H., VEEN, J, BROUWER, E., HUISMAN-DE BROUWER, L., & KOOLEN, J.L. (1968) Residues of chlorinated hydrocarbon insecticides in the North Sea environment. Helgoländer wiss. Meerunters., 17: 375-380.

KORTE, F. (1963) Review of metabolism studies with ^{14}C-labelled insecticides from 1958 to March 1963. Unpublished paper presented at a Toxicological Meeting, New York, 25-27 March.

KORTE, F. (1967) Metabolism of ^{14}C-labelled insecticides in microorganisms, insects, and mammals. Botyu-Kagaku, 32(2): 46-59.

KORTE, F. & STIASNI, M. (1964) [Metabolism of ^{14}C-Telodrin in microorganisms and mosquito larvae.] Ann. Chem., 673: 146-152 (in German).

LAWRENCE, L.J. & CASIDA, J.E. (1984) Interactions of lindane, toxaphene, and cyclodienes with brain-specific t-butylbicyclophosphorothionate receptor. Life Sci., 35: 171-178.

LAYTON, D.W., MALLON, B.J., ROSENBLATT, D.H., & SMALL, M.J. (1987) Deriving allowable daily intakes for systemic toxicants lacking chronic toxicity data. Regul. Toxicol. Pharmacol., 7: 96-112.

MCCASKEY, T.A., STEMP, A.R., LISKA, B.J., & STADELMAN, W.J. (1968) Residues in egg yolks and raw and cooked tissues from laying hens administered selected chlorinated hydrocarbon insecticides. Poultry Sci., 47: 564-569.

MARLOW, R.G., BULL, M.S., & WILLIAMS, S. (1968) Residues of organochlorine insecticides in foodstuffs from Spain, Sittingbourne, Shell International Chemical Company, Ltd (Technical Service Report WKTR.0058.68).

MATHEWS, B.L. (1969) Residues of organochlorine insecticides in foodstuffs from India, Sittingbourne, Shell Research (Report No. WKGR.0102.69).

MATHEWS, B.L. & COLE, E.R. (1966) Residues of Telodrin, methylparathion, and DDT on tobacco from Costa Rica, Sittingbourne, Shell International Chemical Company, Ltd (Technical Service Note 123/66).

MEHROTRA, B.D., BANSAL, S.K., & DESAIAH, D. (1982) Comparative effects of structurally-related cyclodiene pesticides on ATPases. J. appl. Toxicol., 2(6): 278-283.

MOEED, A. (1975) Effects of isobenzan, fensulfothion, and diazinon on invertebrates and microorganisms. N. Z. J. exp. Agric., 3: 181-185.

MOSS, J.A. & HATHWAY, D.E. (1964) Transport of organic compounds in the mammal. Partition of dieldrin and Telodrin between the cellular components and soluble proteins of blood. Biochem. J., 91: 384-393.

MURPHY, M.W. & STANDEN, M.E. (1964) The translocation of Telodrin into potatoes, Sittingbourne, Shell International Chemical Company, Ltd (Technical Memorandum 184/64).

RIBBENS, P.H. (1985) Mortality study of industrial workers exposed to aldrin, dieldrin and endrin. Arch. occup. environ. Health, 56(2): 75-79.

RICHARDSON, A., ROBINSON, J., BUSH, B., & DAVIES, J.M. (1967) Determination of dieldrin (HEOD) in blood. Arch. environ. Health, 14(5): 703-708.

ROBINSON, J. & RICHARDSON, A.R. (1963) The distribution, storage, and elimination of Telodrin in rats fed this insecticide in their diet, Sittingbourne, Shell Research (Report No. R(T)-1-63).

SCHAFER, E.W. & BRUNTON, R.B. (1979) Indicator bird species for toxicity determinations: is the technique usable in test method development? In: Beck, J.R., ed. Vertebrate pest control and management materials, Philadelphia, American Society for Testing and Materials, pp. 157-168 (ASTM STP 680).

SHELL (1963) An episode of pesticide contamination of pasture and dairy products - Isobenzan in Victoria, Australia, in 1963. Melbourne, Shell Chemical Australia (Unpublished report No. 90111501WP5).

SHELL (1964) Telodrin residues. A summary, London, Shell International Chemical Company (Unpublished report).

SPYNU, E.I. (1964) On the toxicology of new organic chloride insecticides obtained by diene synthesis on the basis of hexachlorocyclopentadiene. Gig. Tr. prof. Zabol., 4: 30-35.

SRIVASTAVA, S.C. (1966) The effect of Telodrin on nitrification of ammonia in soil and its implication on nitrogen nutrition of sugarcane. Plant Soil, 25(3): 471-473.

STANDEN, M.E. & ELGAR, K.E. (1965) Telodrin residues in dairy products from Venezuela, Sittingbourne, Shell International Chemical Company, Ltd (Technical Memorandum 36/65).

STEMP, A.R. & LISKA, B.J. (1966) Effects of processing and storage of dairy products on Telodrin and methoxychlor residues. J. diary Sci., **49**: 1006-1008.

STEVENSON, D.E. (1964) The toxicology of Telodrin. Meded. Fac. Landbouwwet. Rijksuniv. Gent, **29**: 1198-1207.

SUZUKI, K., NAGAYOSHI, H., & KASHIWA, T. (1974) The systematic separation and identification of pesticides in the first division. Agric. biol. Chem., **38**(2): 279-285.

THOMPSON, A.R. (1973) Persistence of biological activity of seven insecticides in soil assayed with *Folsomia candida*. J. econ. Entomol., **66**(4): 855-857.

TRUDGILL, P.W. & WIDDUS, R. (1970) Effects of chlorinated insecticides on metabolic processes in bacteria. Biochem. J., **118**: 48-49.

TUINSTRA, L.G.M.TH. & TRAAG, W.A. (1979) Automated glass capillary gas chromatographic analysis of PCB and organochlorine pesticide residues in agricultural products. J. high Resolut. Chromatogr. Chromatogr. Commun., **2**(2): 723-728.

US EPA (1987) Acute toxicity handbook of chemicals to estuarine organisms. Springfield, Virginia, US Department of Commerce, National Technical Information Service (EPA/600/8-87/017).

VAN WIJNEN, J.H. & STIJKEL, A. (1988) Health risk assessment of residents living on harbour sludge. Int. Arch. occup. environ. Health, **61**: 77-87.

VERMA, M.P., BAHGA, H.S., & SONI, B.K. (1967) Effect of prolonged administration of the insecticide Telodrin in poultry. Indian vet. J., **44**: 962-966.

VERSTEEG, J.P.J. & JAGER, K.W. (1973) Long-term occupational exposure to the insecticides aldrin, dieldrin, endrin, and Telodrin. Br. J. ind. Med., **30**: 201-202.

WARE, G.W. & GOOD, E.E. (1967) Effects of insecticides on reproduction in the laboratory mouse. II. Mirex, Telodrin, and DDT. Toxicol. appl. Pharmacol., **10**(1): 54-61.

WEGMAN, R.C.C. & GREVE, P.A. (1980) Halogenated hydrocarbons in Dutch water samples over the years 1969-77. Environ. Sci. Res., **16**: 405-415.

WEGMAN, R.C.C. & HOFSTEE, A.W.M. (1982) Determination of organochlorines in river sediment by capillary gas chromatography. Water Res., **16**: 1265-1272.

WEGMAN, R.C.C., HOFSTEE, A.W.M., & GREVE, P.A. (1981) Uptake of organochlorines by plants growing on river and basin sediment. Meded. Fac. Landbouwwet. Rijksuniv. Gent, **46**(1): 359-365.

WORDEN, A.N. (1969) Toxicity of Telodrin. Toxicol. appl. Pharmacol., **14**: 556-573.

ZAVON, M.R. (1961) Toxicology and pharmacology of Telodrin insecticide (compound SD 4402), Cincinnati, Ohio, The Kettering Laboratory (Unpublished report).

RESUME ET EVALUATION; CONCLUSIONS ET RECOMMANDATIONS

1. Résumé et évaluation

Autant qu'on sache, l'isobenzan, un insecticide organochloré n'a été fabriqué que pendant la période 1958-1965. Plusieurs années après, on puisait toujours sur les stocks existants. A l'heure actuelle, les seules sources importantes d'exposition sont vraisemblablement les sites de décharge initiaux de déchets industriels ou les boues de dragage provenant de sédiments contaminés.

Une fois épandu sur le sol, la majeure partie de l'isobenzan disparaît rapidement. Après quoi, la fraction restante se décompose beaucoup plus lentement. Elle persiste dans le sol de deux à sept ans selon la nature de celui-ci. Au laboratoire, l'isobenzan se décompose dans les eaux de surface en l'espace de quelques semaines lorsqu'il est exposé à la lumière naturelle ou artificielle.

Le sol, les eaux souterraines et superficielles provenant des polders constitués de sédiments contaminés par des organochlorés, notamment des dérivés cyclodiéniques, contenaient encore plusieurs années après, de faibles résidus d'isobenzan. En 1979-1980, on n'a pas détecté d'isobenzan (limite de détection 0,01 mg/kg de poids sec) dans les sédiments des cours d'eau des Pays-Bas. Après traitement du sol, les résidus qui subsistent sur les récoltes sont généralement faibles (inférieurs à 0,05 mg/kg de végétaux), mais on peut en trouver des quantités plus fortes sur certaines racines (jusqu'à 0,2 mg/kg dans les carottes). Des enquêtes de type "panier de la ménagère" effectuées lorsqu'on utilisait de l'isobenzan en agriculture, n'ont pas permis de déceler de résidus dans les denrées contrôlées (moins de 0,01 mg/kg).

Chaque fois qu'on a laissé paître des bovins dans des pâturages traités par de l'isobenzan, on a constaté que les produits laitiers obtenus contenaient des résidus de cet insecticide. C'est ainsi que dans deux échantillons de beurre, on a trouvé 0,07 et 0,15 mg d'isobenzan par kg de produit, les concentrations dans le lait entier allant de 0,005 à 0,07 mg/kg. Le lait en poudre n'en contenait toutefois que 0,005 mg/kg. Lors du traitement industriel des

Résumé et Evaluation; Conclusions et Recommandations

produits laitiers, plus de 50% du résidu disparaît selon le type de traitement.

On ne dispose d'aucune donnée sur les quantités d'isobenzan présentes dans le sang ou les tissus adipeux de la population générale. Des travailleurs exposés à l'isobenzan lors de la fabrication ou de la formulation de cet insecticide, présentaient des taux sanguins (sang total) allant jusqu'à 0,041 mg/litre. Dans les échantillons de sang total prélevés sur des personnes vivant à proximité d'une unité de production, la concentration d'isobenzan était inférieure à la limite de détection (0,001 mg/litre).

L'isobenzan est facilement résorbé par la paroi du tube digestif et il passe dans le sang sans modification. Il se forme des métabolites hydrophiles et notamment une lactone. L'isobenzan s'accumule dans les tissus et les organes des rats et des chiens selon l'ordre: graisses > foie = muscle > cerveau > sang. Les concentrations tissulaires chez les rattes sont généralement plus faibles que chez les rats, spécialement dans les graisses. La demi-vie biologique dans le tissu adipeux était ainsi de 10,9 jours chez les rats et de 16,6 jours chez les rattes. Chez un chiot femelle dont le sang contenait 0,09 mg d'isobenzan par litre, on a observé des convulsions 15 jours après la naissance. L'animal n'avait été nourri qu'avec le lait de sa mère, une chienne Beagle à qui l'on avait fait absorber de l'isobenzan et dont le lait en contenait 0,7 mg/litre. Des effets analogues sur les petits ont été observés lors d'une étude de reproduction sur le rat. Chez la vache, l'isobenzan est excrété dans le lait.

Les larves de moustiques et les champignons terricoles métabolisent l'isobenzan de la même manière que les vertébrés, notamment sous forme de lactone. L'isobenzan est très persistant dans l'environnement et s'accumule dans les organismes vivants. Il est extrêmement toxique pour les poissons, les crevettes et les oiseaux. Aux Pays-Bas, pays où l'on fabriquait l'isobenzan, on a trouvé des résidus dans des oeufs de sternes vivant sur la côte hollandaise qui atteignaient 0,45 mg/kg (moyenne, 0,09 mg/kg). Dans les moules et le poisson, les résidus moyens étaient de 0,05 mg/kg en 1965. Dans les parcelles traitées par de l'isobenzan à raison de 2 kg/ha, on a constaté une réduction du nombre de lombrics. Il y avait réduction de la nitrification avec accroissement corrélatif de l'azote minéral dans les sols traités par l'isobenzan à raison d'1 kg/ha; en revanche, les études en laboratoire n'ont mis en évidence aucun effet sur la nitrification à des doses correspondant à 250 g/ha.

L'isobenzan présente une forte toxicité aiguë pour les mammifères, que ce soit par la voie orale ou par la voie percutanée. Le mode d'action de l'isobenzan consiste en une stimulation excessive du système nerveaux central conduisant à des convulsions. La toxicité aiguë des diverses formulations d'isobenzan correspond à la proportion de matière active.

L'isobenzan n'est pas irritant pour la peau mais certaines de ses formulations peuvent l'être.

Des études limitées à court et à long terme, au cours desquelles on a administré par voie orale de l'isobenzan à des souris, à des rats et à des chiens, ont montré que ce composé pouvait induire des lésions histologiques au niveau du foie, du type de celles qu'on observe classiquement avec les organochlorés. Une étude de longue durée sur des rats a permis de déterminer que la dose sans effet observable était de 5 mg/kg de nourriture (soit l'équivalent de 0,25 mg/kg de poids corporel). Chez le chien, la dose sans effet nocif observable, déterminée à la suite d'une étude de deux ans, était de 0,025 mg/kg de poids corporel.

Une étude de reproduction portant sur une génération de rats a montré que la dose sans effet nocif observable était de 0,1 mg/kg de nourriture (soit l'équivalent de 0,05 mg/kg de poids corporel. A la dose de 1 mg/kg de nourriture (soit l'équivalent de 0,05 mg/kg de poids corporel), il y a eu réduction de la survie des ratons.

Aucune étude de tératogénicité ni de mutagénicité n'a été rapportée.

Une étude de deux ans sur des rats (administration par voie orale) et une étude sur des souris n'ont pas permis de mettre en évidence un pouvoir cancérogène quelconque, mais ces études n'étaient pas adaptées à une telle évaluation.

La base de données toxicologiques sur l'isobenzan est incomplète. En général on estime que, d'après les critères actuels, les données sont d'une qualité médiocre et sont en tous cas insuffisantes pour permettre une évaluation du risque que ce composé présente pour la santé humaine ou l'environnement.

Les données concernant l'exposition humaine se limitent à des études effectuées sur des travailleurs d'une usine hollandaise qui étaient employés à la fabrication et à la formulation d'isobenzan et d'insecticides cyclodiéniques apparentés. Aucun cas d'irritation cutanée n'a été signalé. Dans plusieurs cas d'intoxication, on a observé des convulsions mais les anomalies du tracé électroencéphalographique étaient réversibles. Le seuil limite d'intoxication (pour les convulsions), a été estimé à 0,015 mg d'isobenzan par litre de sang et la demi-vie biologique de ce composé dans le sang humain est, semble-t-il, de l'ordre de 2,8 années.

2. Conclusions et recommandations

L'isobenzan est extrêmement toxique et très persistant. Les données dont on dispose sur le danger qu'il représente sont incomplètes mais néanmoins suffisantes pour montrer que ce danger est réel pour les personnes qui le manipulent ainsi que pour l'environnement, de sorte qu'il faut éviter toute contamination humaine ou environnementale qui résulterait de l'utilisation de ce produit comme insecticide ou autre.

RESUMEN Y EVALUACION; CONCLUSIONES Y RECOMENDACIONES

1. Resumen y evaluación

Según los datos de que se dispone, el isobenzano, un insecticida organoclorado, sólo se fabricó durante el periodo 1958-1965. Durante los años siguientes se utilizaron las existencias almacenadas. En la actualidad, se cree que las únicas fuentes importantes de exposición son los lugares donde originalmente se evacuaron los desechos industriales o los materiales dragados de sedimentos contaminados.

Cuando se aplica el isobenzano al suelo, se produce una rápida pérdida inicial; después, el resto del compuesto se degrada mucho más despacio. Persiste en el suelo durante 2 a 7 años, según el tipo de suelo. En condiciones de laboratorio, el isobenzano se descompone en las aguas de superficie en pocas semanas cuando se expone a la luz natural o artificial.

El suelo, las aguas subterráneas y las aguas superficiales de pólders construidos con sedimentos contaminados por sustancias organocloradas, inclusive compuestos de ciclodieno clorado, aún contenían pequeños residuos de isobenzano algunos años después. En 1979-1980, no se detectó isobenzano (límite de detección: 0,01 mg/kg de peso seco) en el sedimento de ríos de los Países Bajos. Tras el tratamiento del suelo, los residuos en las cosechas suelen ser bajos (menos de 0,05 mg/kg de cosecha), pero pueden encontrarse concentraciones superiores en algunos tubérculos (hasta 0,2 mg/kg en zanahorias). En las encuestas de mercado realizadas durante la época de uso agrícola del isobenzano no se detectaron residuos en los alimentos analizados (menos de 0,01 mg/kg).

En los productos lácteos procedentes de ganado que se alimentó en pastos tratados con isobenzano se encontraron residuos del insecticida. Dos muestras de mantequilla contenían 0,07 y 0,15 mg de isobenzano/kg de producto, mientras que los niveles en la leche entera fueron de 0,005 mg/kg a 0,07 mg/kg. En la leche deshidratada, no obstante, se encontraron sólo 0,005 mg/kg. Durante la elaboración de los productos lácteos se perdía hasta el 50% del residuo, según el tipo de tratamiento.

No se dispone de datos sobre los niveles de isobenzano en la sangre o el tejido adiposo de la población general. Los operarios expuestos al isobenzano en las plantas de fabricación y elaboración presentaron niveles medios en sangre entera de hasta 0,041 mg/litro. En muestras de sangre entera procedente de personas que vivían en las proximidades de una de las plantas, la concentración de isobenzano estaba por debajo del límite de detección (0,001 mg/litro).

El isobenzano es absorbido rápidamente a través de la pared gastrointestinal y es transportado por la sangre sin alteraciones. Se forman metabolitos hidrófilos de los que se ha identificado uno, la lactona de isobenzano. El isobenzano se acumula en los tejidos y los órganos de ratas y perros en el orden siguiente: grasa > hígado = músculo > cerebro > sangre. Las concentraciones tisulares en las hembras de rata son en general superiores a las que aparecen en los machos, sobre todo en la grasa. En la rata se determinó que la semivida biológica en la grasa del organismo es de 10,9 días en los machos y 16,6 días en las hembras. En un cachorro hembra de perro, cuya sangre contenía 0,09 mg de isobenzano/litro, se observaron convulsiones a los 15 días del nacimiento. El cachorro sólo se había alimentado de leche de su madre, una Beagle a la que se había administrado isobenzano y cuya leche contenía 0,7 mg/litro. En un estudio de reproducción en ratas se observaron efectos similares en las crías. Las vacas excretan isobenzano con la leche.

Las larvas de mosquito y los hongos del suelo metabolizan el isobenzano del mismo modo que los vertebrados, dando lactona de isobenzano como metabolito.

El isobenzano es muy persistente en el medio ambiente y se bioacumula. Es sumamente tóxico para los peces, los camarones y las aves. En los Países Bajos, país en el que se fabricaba el isobenzano, los residuos encontrados en los huevos de golondrinas de mar de las costas holandesas ascendieron a 0,45 mg/kg (promedio: 0,09 mg/kg), mientras que el promedio de residuos encontrados en mejillones y peces fue de 0,05 mg/kg en 1965. Se observó una disminución del número de lombrices en terrenos tratados con isobenzano a razón de 2 kg/ha. Se redujo la nitrificación, con el consiguiente aumento del nitrógeno inorgánico, en los suelos tratados con isobenzano sobre el terreno a razón de 1 kg/ha, si bien en estudios de laboratorio no se demostró efecto alguno en la nitrificación con dosis equivalentes a 250 g/ha.

La toxicidad aguda del isobenzano para los mamíferos es elevada por las vías oral y percutánea. La forma de acción de su toxicidad es la sobreestimulación del sistema nervioso central, que da lugar a convulsiones. La toxicidad aguda de las preparaciones de isobenzano refleja el porcentaje de ingrediente activo presente.

Aunque el isobenzano no irrita la piel, algunos productos preparados a partir de él pueden causar irritación.

En estudios limitados a corto y largo plazo de administración oral realizados en ratones, ratas y perros se ha demostrado que el isobenzano puede provocar en el hígado cambios histológicos que reponden al tipo clásico de intoxicación por compuestos organoclorados. En un estudio realizado a largo plazo en ratas, se determinó un nivel efectos sin observados de 5 mg/kg de dieta (equivalente a 0,25 mg/kg de peso corporal), y en un estudio en perros de dos años de duración se determinó un nivel sin observación de efectos adversos de 0,025 mg/kg de peso corporal.

En un estudio de reproducción en una generación de ratas se obtuvo un nivel sin efectos adversos observados de 0,1 mg/kg de dieta (equivalente a 0,05 mg/kg de peso corporal). Con un nivel de 1 mg/kg de dieta (equivalente a 0,05 mg/kg de peso corporal) disminuyó la supervivencia de las crías.

No se han comunicado estudios sobre la teratogenicidad ni la mutagenicidad del compuesto.

No se observó potencial carcinogénico en un estudio de administración oral a ratas durante dos años ni en un estudio de administración oral a ratones, pero esos estudios no eran apropiados para evaluar la carcinogenicidad.

La base de datos toxicológicos correspondiente al isobenzano es incompleta. En general, actualmente se considera que la calidad de los datos es mediocre e insuficiente para evaluar los riesgos que representa para la salud humana o el medio ambiente.

Los datos sobre personas expuestas se limitan a estudios realizados en trabajadores de una fábrica de los Países Bajos durante la fabricación y la elaboración de preparaciones de isobenzano y otros insecticidas de ciclodieno clorado afines. No se comunicaron casos de irritación cutánea. En varios casos de intoxicación, se produjeron convulsiones pero los cambios del trazado electroencefalográfico resultaron ser reversibles. El nivel umbral de intoxicación (en el caso de las convulsiones) se estimó en 0,015 mg de isobenzano/litro de sangre, y se calculó que la semivida biológica del isobenzano en la sangre humana es del orden de 2,8 años.

2. Conclusiones y recomendaciones

El isobenzano es sumamente tóxico y muy persistente. La información de que se dispone sobre los riegos del isobenzano es incompleta, pero, aún así, basta para indicar que el riesgo que supone para los que lo manipulan y para el medio ambiente es tan elevado que no debería permitirse la exposición humana o del medio ambiente a esta sustancia, ya sea utilizada como insecticida o para cualquier otro fin.

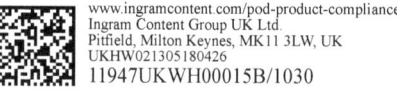

www.ingramcontent.com/pod-product-compliance
Ingram Content Group UK Ltd.
Pitfield, Milton Keynes, MK11 3LW, UK
UKHW021305180426
11947UKWH00015B/1030